Y0-EIB-919

WITHDRAWN

Carnegie Mellon

HEALTH CARE POLICY IN THE UNITED STATES

edited by

JOHN G. BRUHN
PENNSYLVANIA STATE
UNIVERSITY-HARRISBURG

A GARLAND SERIES

Health Care Policy in the United States
John G. Bruhn, editor

WHO CARES FOR POOR PEOPLE?

PHYSICIANS, MEDICAID, AND MARGINALITY

MARGARET M. HYNES

GARLAND PUBLISHING, INC.
A MEMBER OF THE TAYLOR & FRANCIS GROUP
NEW YORK & LONDON / 1998

H Copyright © 1998 Margaret M. Hynes

Library of Congress Cataloging-in-Publication Data

Hynes, Margaret M., 1953–
    Who cares forpoor people? : physicians, medicaid, and
marginality / Margaret M. Hynes.
        p.   cm. — (Health care policy in the United States)
    Includes bibliographical references and index.
    ISBN 0-8153-3045-6 (alk. paper)
    1. Medicaid. 2. Physicians—United States. 3. Occupational
prestige—United States. 4. Poor—Medical care—United States.
I. Title. II. Series: Health care policy in the United States (New
York, N.Y.)
RA412.4.H96 1998
362.1'086'9420973—dc21

                                                        98-28108

Printed on acid-free, 250-year-life paper
Manufactured in the United States of America

Dedicated to the memory of my parents
Helen Gadomski Hynes, R.N. and
Thomas Vincent Hynes II, M.D.

Contents

Tables and Figures

Acknowledgments

Thoughts of my childhood household, an extension of my father's medical practice, were close by as I developed this book. I am grateful to my parents, Thomas Vincent and Helen Gadomski Hynes, for the compassionate humanity with which they lived and worked. In the pre-Medicaid era, as a solo medical practitioner my father provided a great deal of primary care to low-income patients at little or no cost. My parents oftentimes welcomed less fortunate patients into our home for a cup of tea or soup, some conversation, and occasionally, a bed for the night. As I prepared the current version of this manuscript in the year following the death of my mother Helen, I was reminded over and over again in myriad ways of her kind and generous influence on me. I feel fortunate to have had her for so many years in my life. I am also grateful to my older siblings, Tom, John, Mike, Ed, Pat, Mary, Veronica, and Monica, who encouraged me to work and educate myself, as well as to the many members of my extended family, particularly Mary Nikkel Doyle, Jane Bradley, and Jan Raymond, for their guidance and inspiration over many years.

   This study uses data from a national survey of physicians, nurses, and AIDS. I am grateful to the Agency for Health Care Policy and Research for providing funding for that study (AHCPR Grant Number 5 R01 HS06359). I would also like to thank the many people who assisted me in this project including Kristi Long, Chuck Bartelt and Rebecca Wipfler of Garland Publishing for their advice in preparation of the manuscript; Chau Trinh for her assistance in preparation of the bibliography; Chin-Lin Tseng for her detailed and thoughtful comments on parts of the manuscript; and my sister Pat Hynes who, despite her own demanding schedule, found time to comment constructively on my work page by page.

An earlier version of this manuscript benefited from comments by faculty members of the Columbia University School of Public Health— John Colombotos, Jack Elinson, Mary Clare Lennon, Peter Messeri and Anne Reisinger. I am particularly grateful to Peter Messeri for numerous conversations regarding the conceptual and analytic frameworks for this study. Above all, I owe my deep gratitude to John Colombotos who graciously allowed me to use data from his national study and commented extensively on both earlier and later versions of this manuscript. Any mistakes in this work are entirely my own.

Finally, I am deeply indebted to the Asencio family—Juan Eliseo, Adelaida Sánchez, Eliseo, Fabio Silva, and Marysol—for their day to day care of me during my work on this book. In particular, I remember Adelaida, who passed away after a long illness, for her courage. Lastly, I thank my dear Marysol for her steadfast support throughout this process from beginning to end.

Who Cares for Poor People?

I

Introduction

Medicaid, the federally funded and state administered program of medical assistance for poor Americans, is one component of the United States' pluralistic health care system. While the majority of Americans receive health care coverage through employer-based private insurance, some segments of the population are covered through publicly funded programs such as Medicaid, for low-income families and the disabled, and Medicare, for the elderly. A steadily growing portion of the American population has no medical insurance. This segment, not covered by either the private or the public systems, includes part-time wage earners and small business and independent workers.

A national plan of universal health coverage has, at various times throughout American history, reached prominence as an important issue for public action, most recently in 1993–1994 during the Clinton Administration. Historical factors, such as a national ethos of personal freedom and minimal government interference, as well as entrenched interests within the government and the medical and health care industries are reasons cited for the failure of a comprehensive national health program (Fry et al. 1995; Navarro 1995). It is within the context of this larger national health care debate that any discussion regarding the health care of poor Americans takes place.

Medicaid was enacted by Congress as Title XIX of the Social Security Act of 1965 with two principal aims: to make medical services available to people who would otherwise be unable to afford them; and to encourage the utilization of those services in the private office-based sector, "the mainstream" of American medicine. Medicaid is widely recognized as

3

having closed some gaps between the poor and nonpoor in access to care and as having established a safety net for poor and disabled Americans needing long-term care services (Spiegel 1975; Iglehart 1993; Rowland 1994, 1995). More than 35 million Americans received health care coverage through Medicaid in 1995 (Kaiser Commission on the Future of Medicaid 1997).

Since the enactment of Medicaid legislation, however, public policy initiatives concerning the health of poor Americans and their access to medical care have been the subject of considerable scrutiny (Stevens and Stevens 1974; Institute of Medicine 1981; Starr 1986; Garber 1989; Cornelius 1991; Iglehart 1993; Rowland 1994, 1995). Research has shown that many Medicaid patients have limited access to primary health care outside hospital emergency departments. Policy analysts have cited barriers to access as a major indication that the restructuring of Medicaid is long overdue (Medicaid Access Study Group 1994).

With the collapse of comprehensive national health initiatives in 1994, legislative proposals aimed at controlling soaring health care costs targeted the Medicaid program. Although managed care has become a major vehicle for the restructuring of Medicaid in the 1990s, its impact nationwide on improving access for diverse subgroups within the Medicaid population is still uncertain.

The present study examines one component of access to health care —the variables related to physician participation in the federal Medicaid program—and develops a theoretical framework in which to understand its significance. Previous studies, examining only office-based physicians, suggest that economic self-interest and physician shortages in low-income areas are important factors related to their participation in this federally-funded program.

In contrast to previous studies, this study examines physicians in both office and institutional settings to investigate who, in fact, cares for Medicaid patients as well as the social variables related to their participation. It also examines whether the physicians most likely to care for Medicaid patients are those who have traditionally been "marginal" to the profession. "Marginal physicians" are those who are less "credentialed" (that is, foreign medical school graduates and physicians without board certification) and those who historically have been discriminated against in the larger society, such as nonwhites[1] and women.

Marginality is a social condition associated with long-standing social and economic barriers and is the result of a process of formal and/or informal discrimination. Individuals possessing less desirable marginal social statuses find that opportunities for advancement within the medical profession are limited. Marginality in the medical profession results from disadvantages stemming from the gradual accumulation of marginal statuses.

This study employs a secondary analysis of data from a 1990 national survey of physicians and nurses regarding HIV/AIDS[2] to explore the marginality thesis. Data for 958 physicians included information about their social and professional backgrounds as well as the extent of their participation in Medicaid.

The book is organized as follows:

Chapter Two reviews the previous empirical studies related to physician participation in the Medicaid program since its inception in the 1960s as well as the conceptual frameworks used to analyze the phenomenon. It addresses government policies, physician supply, and physician ideology in relationship to Medicaid participation.

Chapter Three explores the concept of marginality and "the marginal man" in the sociological literature. It also reviews the empirical literature related to marginal groups in the medical profession.

Chapter Four describes the data sources, methods, and measurements used for this study's analysis. It also analyzes nonresponse bias and differences of respondents by phase and interview mode.

Chapter Five presents descriptive findings of the study. Physicians are profiled by their social statuses, professional statuses, and practice characteristics as well as the patterned ways in which these statuses and characteristics overlap. The relationships among physicians' social statuses and practice characteristics and their political and professional ideologies are also discussed.

Chapter Six presents analytic findings of this study including a discussion of factors related to physician participation in Medicaid. The relative importance of physicians' social statuses, professional statuses and characteristics, and ideology in explaining their participation in Medicaid is also discussed.

Chapter Seven provides a summary of conclusions of this study, situating them in the context of Medicaid reform in the 1990s. It also suggests important areas for further research and outlines some implications for public policy.

NOTES

1. In this study, the system of racial/ethnic classifications issued by the U.S. Office of Management and Budget in 1975 will be used. The term "minorities" will be used in place of "nonwhite" to identify those whose racial category is American Indian, Asian and Pacific Islander, African American, and white/nonwhite Hispanics. The term "white" will identify all other nonminority individuals.

2. Colombotos, John, Peter Messeri, Marianne Burgunder McConnell, Jack Elinson, Donald Gemson, and Margaret Hynes, Columbia University School of Public Health. 1995. *Physicians, Nurses, and AIDS: Findings From a National Study*. Rockville, MD: Agency for Health Care Policy and Research; 1995. Available from: NTIS, Springfield, VA; PB95-129185.

This research was supported by the Agency for Health Care Policy and Research under AHCPR Grant Number 5 R01 HS06359.

II

Physician Participation in Medicaid

BACKGROUND

Since the 1970s, evidence has shown that private office-based physicians have either limited or withdrawn their participation in Medicaid programs (Jones and Hamburger 1976; Garner, Liao, and Sharpe 1979; Davidson 1982; Perloff, Kletke, and Neckerman 1986; Mitchell 1991). The statistics have varied by year, state, and the exact measure of participation; however, the trend away from office-based physician participation has been unmistakable.

Numerous recent studies indicate that many Medicaid patients lack access to primary care physicians and, by default, use hospital emergency rooms (Pane, Farner, and Salness 1991; Baker, Stevens, and Brook 1991; Bindman et al. 1991; Shesser et al. 1993; Grumbach, Keane, and Bindman 1993; Medicaid Access Study Group 1994). This phenomenon of "site-shifting" by Medicaid recipients has been documented in analyses of utilization and site-of-visit patterns nationwide (Long, Settle, and Stuart 1986). The concern is echoed by policy analysts who have pointed to the inappropriate use of hospital emergency room departments by Medicaid patients as a source of skyrocketing health care costs (Kusserow 1992a). According to a study by the U.S. General Accounting Office the number of visits by Medicaid patients to hospital emergency departments increased by 34 percent between 1985 and 1990 (Nadel 1993).

Cohen's analysis of 1987 data from the National Medical Expenditure Survey supports the idea that better access to office-based physician care

9

is associated with better health outcomes. He found that Medicaid patients with an office-based physician as a usual source of care were five percent less likely to be admitted to a hospital than were those who used an emergency room or hospital outpatient department as a usual source of care (Cohen 1993). Other analysts such as Fossett, Choi, and Peterson (1991) argue, however, that because there is a severe shortage of office-based physicians in urban areas, the most convenient and accessible alternative for Medicaid patients in urban areas may be hospital outpatient clinics:

> As a result of declining admissions, many urban teaching hospitals are currently seeking ambulatory training sites as an alternative to traditional inpatient sites. Hospital-linked clinics staffed primarily by residents, with hours and appointment systems that more closely parallel those of emergency rooms, might provide a means of reducing inappropriate use of outpatient facilities (Fossett et al.1991: 975).

Major efforts to reform Medicaid in the 1990s have relied on managed care approaches at the state level. By January 1995, all states except Alaska were experimenting with various models in an attempt to control escalating costs (Grogan 1997). Medicaid patients have been rapidly enrolled in a variety of managed care plans. In 1990, less than nine percent of the U.S. Medicaid population was enrolled in managed care compared to 40 percent in 1997 (*Managed Care Week* October 3, 1994; Rosenbaum 1997).

Managed care aims to restructure health care financing and delivery systems primarily through the use of a "gatekeeper," usually a primary care physician who, ideally, incorporates preventive health practices that are cost-effective and improve patient health outcomes. In theory, managed care reduces financial barriers to physicians' participation in Medicaid by paying them on a capitation basis.

It is possible that Medicaid managed care will increase provider participation and thereby decrease Medicaid patients' use of emergency departments for non-urgent care. A major impediment to the successful implementation of Medicaid managed care, however, is the shortage of primary care physicians in low-income neighborhoods. This chapter first examines prior research in three areas: office-based physicians' participation in Medicaid, physician supply in low-income neighborhoods, and physician ideology and its relationship to social and professional characteristics and attitudes. Based on this prior research, I then summarize a set of hypotheses to explain physician participation in Medicaid and describe a causal model and conceptual framework for the data analyzed in this study.

REVIEW OF PRIOR RESEARCH

Economic and Sociological Theories of Self-interest

Since the 1970s, numerous studies have investigated factors influencing office-based physicians' decisionmaking regarding acceptance of Medicaid patients (Jones and Hamburger 1976; Hadley 1978; Sloan, Cromwell, and Mitchell 1978; Held, Manheim, and Wooldrige 1978; Mitchell and Cromwell 1980; Mitchell 1983; Davidson 1982; Mitchell and Shurman 1984; Perloff, Kletke, and Neckerman 1987a; Fossett and Peterson 1989; Fossett, Perloff, Peterson, and Kletke 1990). The analytical model guiding most of this research is the economic two-market theory developed by Sloan et al. (1978), which asserts that physicians have two markets—one private and the other public—in which to sell their services. In the private market the physician sets the prices, whereas in the public market the physician accepts a set payment. Reimbursement in the private market tends to be more lucrative; therefore, according to this economic model, physicians will attempt to take patients in the private non-Medicaid market before accepting patients in the public Medicaid market. The extent to which physicians participate in either of these two markets is a function of four factors: the demand for physician services in each market, the supply of physicians competing for patients in each market, the costs of providing services in each market, and the revenue gained in each market (Sloan et al. 1978).

A sociological theory emphasizing professional autonomy in clinical decisionmaking complements the economic theory in explaining office-based physician participation in Medicaid (Anderson and Lyden 1963; Freidson 1970). It suggests that physicians' willingness to participate in Medicaid is directly related to the amount of clinical discretion they feel they have in practicing medicine in each of the two markets. Historically, the public market in the United States has tended to offer physicians less autonomy in their clinical decisionmaking than the private market and would therefore be considered less desirable by office-based physicians.

There are two underlying assumptions of the economic and sociological theories: first, physicians will always choose positions within the medical marketplace that offer them greater financial reward and autonomy; and second, since the marketplace is competitive, some physicians will be "losers" and thereby forced to take more patients in the less desirable public market. More than two decades of studies (Kavaler 1969; Jones and Hamburger 1976; Mitchell and Cromwell 1980; Fairbrother et al. 1995) have demonstrated that there is a distinctive group of office-based physicians who are most likely to care for Medicaid patients. Foreign medical school graduates[1] and physicians who are not board-certified are overrepresented among office-based physicians with high Medicaid caseloads. These physicians are considered less competitive within the framework of the economic model because they are less credentialed (Sloan et al. 1978: 133).

Government Policies Related to Economic Incentives

State government policies affect office-based physicians' decisions to participate in Medicaid (The Physician Payment Review Commission 1990; 1991). Federal laws have given states wide latitude in determining eligibility and reimbursement guidelines and processing of claims for Medicaid. Variations in state Medicaid programs have been analyzed by numerous researchers (Davidson 1978, 1982; Hanson 1984; Rowland, Lyons, and Edwards 1988; Schwartz, Colby, and Reisinger 1991) who contend that low fees, payment delays, and complexity of claims forms in some states contribute to office-based physicians' reluctance to treat

Medicaid patients. The Omnibus Budget Reconciliation Act of 1989 directed the Physician Payment Review Commission (PPRC) to examine the adequacy of physician payment under Medicaid. In 1990, the Commission surveyed state Medicaid programs on physician fees, payment methods, and physician participation and found that wide variation exists among states in the level of Medicaid fees relative to other payers. It also confirmed earlier analyses indicating that Medicaid pays physicians considerably less than Medicare, which, in turn, pays substantially less than private insurers. It is estimated that, on average, private insurers pay 40 to 50 percent more than Medicare, which typically pays 30 percent more than Medicaid (*The New York Times* March 9, 1993).

The 1991 PPRC Commission Report noted that when other payers offer higher rates than Medicaid, office-based physicians are less likely to serve Medicaid patients; however, it observed, "Medicaid fees appear to have no effect on the proportion of Medicaid beneficiaries receiving services, the number of services received, or the probability of contact with a physician." It concluded that "fee levels...do appear to affect the site in which services are received. In areas where Medicaid fees were only half as high as Medicare's, more visits took place in settings such as outpatient departments, emergency rooms, health department clinics, and community and migrant health centers" (PPRC 1991: 296).

A 1991 study of county level Medicaid claims data from the state of Illinois found, however, that there was "little evidence that outpatient care substitutes for care by (office-based) physicians or that raising physician fees would reduce inappropriate outpatient usage by Medicaid patients" (Fossett et al. 1991: 964). Because severe shortages of office-based physicians exist in low-income urban areas, it appears that outpatient and emergency care do not displace office-based physician care (Fossett et al. 1991: 965).

Issues Related to the Physician Supply

Evidence suggests that primary care physicians, in contrast to specialists, tend to draw the majority of their patients from areas surrounding their practices (Kletke and Marder 1987). This tendency is more pronounced among lower-income groups in urban areas compared to higher-income groups (Acton 1976; Dutton 1978). In light of these findings, policy analysts have raised concerns about shortages of primary care physicians in urban areas and the implications for health status of the urban poor (USDHHS 1990b).

Medicaid researchers in the 1980s began to observe a trend which was apparently inconsistent with the economic two-market model, namely, that at the county level of analysis, a greater physician supply is associated with a decrease in the extent of physician participation in Medicaid (Perloff et al. 1986; Fossett and Peterson 1989). (The two-market model posits that physicians compete for patients and a greater supply of physicians results in greater competition for all patients and thereby greater participation in Medicaid.) In a longitudinal study of office-based pediatricians' participation in state Medicaid programs, Perloff et al. (1986) found that this relationship strengthened over time. In 1978, a greater provider supply was not significantly associated with less Medicaid participation; however, by 1983, it had become significant. Perloff et al. point out that this finding suggests an increased physician supply is not related to greater Medicaid participation among office-based pediatricians, but that future investigations into this apparent trend would better interpret this finding.

Fossett and Peterson's (1989) research also points to the importance of physician supply factors in understanding participation in Medicaid. Their analysis of 1985 county level data in Illinois indicates that office-based physicians tend to have either "mostly private" or "mostly public" clientele practices due, plausibly, to residential segregation. They observe that residential segregation between Medicaid and private patients and high physician practice costs may discourage physician participation in urban areas. This fact offsets the effects of competition among primary care physicians that one would expect to see in a two-market framework. It is quite possible that this either-or tendency is also enhanced by discriminatory behavior of physicians who hesitate to mix practices fearing that the stigmatizing effect of Medicaid patients will cause a loss in private patients. They also note:

> These considerations suggest strongly that the degree of residential segregation between Medicaid and private patients is a major determinant of the ability and willingness of physicians to expand the Medicaid share of their practices. In residentially segregated areas, only physicians located in or very close to lower-income areas or in areas readily accessible by public transportation can expand the Medicaid portion of their practices easily. Physicians whose practices are geographically less accessible are likely to experience more difficulty in attracting Medicaid patients because of the extended travel time involved in seeking care (Fossett and Peterson 1989:388).

This analysis gains further support by Fossett, Perloff, Peterson, and Kletke's (1990) study of Chicago pediatricians' participation in Medicaid, which found severe shortages of private, office-based physicians working in poverty areas where the majority of Medicaid patients reside. Their research suggests that access to medical care will not be improved by policy decisions (such as expanded Medicaid eligibility and increased provider reimbursement) alone:

> Access to maternity care in these areas is constrained by lack of physicians rather than by lack of Medicaid participation...Expanding Medicaid eligibility or increasing Medicaid reimbursement...(is) unlikely to have any effect on access to care in Chicago's poorest areas...since many, if not most, women are already Medicaid eligible and almost all physicians already accept very large numbers of Medicaid patients (Fossett et al. 1990: 112).

Perloff et al. also concluded that, from 1978 to 1983, the impact of state policy factors on physician participation in Medicaid "diminished over time, while the influence of changes in physician supply...increased" (1986: 749).

Physician Ideology

Some studies of office-based physicians' participation in Medicaid have attempted to assess the role of physician attitudes related to professional autonomy[2] and social welfare issues.[3] "Ideology" may be viewed as a constellation of interrelated attitudes comprising a broader social outlook. Political ideology, for example, may be conceptualized as a set of attitudes regarding political party, social liberalism, and economic-welfare issues.

Perloff et al. (1987a) found that, in 1983, office-based pediatricians not participating in Medicaid were less liberal in their political "social welfare" attitudes than participating pediatricians, but that these attitudes were not significantly related to their extent of participation. That is, among participating pediatricians, those with fewer Medicaid patients were no less liberal than those with greater numbers of Medicaid patients.

In their analysis of fee-for-service private practice physicians, Sloan et al. (1978) also found that greater Medicaid participation was positively associated with liberal "social welfare" attitudes. Physicians who strongly agreed with the statement "It is the responsibility of society, through its government, to provide everyone with the best available medical care, whether he can afford it or not" had, on average, 3.5 percent more Medicaid patients in their practice than those who strongly disagreed. Although statistically significant, this construct alone explained very little of the variation in Medicaid participation. Sloan et al. therefore concluded that physicians' political views were relatively unimportant compared with concrete economic incentives in explaining their decisions to participate in Medicaid.

Sloan et al. (1978) included a second statement regarding physician autonomy ("There are too many controls on the medical profession that interfere with taking care of patients...") but found that there was little variation among participating and nonparticipating physicians. The vast majority of physicians (58 percent of participants and 60 percent of nonparticipants) agreed strongly with this statement.

It can be argued that, on the contrary, physicians' ideology is quite important in understanding their participation in Medicaid, but that previous studies lack well-developed measures of physician ideology or that their analyses have not attempted to explain important social dimensions of physicians' choices. Colombotos has examined physician attitudes toward political, socioeconomic, and health care issues emphasizing the influence of early and later sources of socialization on physician ideology (Colombotos 1969; Colombotos and Kirchner 1986). Using data from Colombotos' national study of physicians and social change, Sudit (1987) found that medical students' attitudes toward national health insurance were influenced by their ideology as well as economic self-interest. Both Colombotos and Sudit demonstrate the relevance of various dimensions of physician ideology in understanding physicians' attitudes toward a variety of health care issues.

Colombotos and Kirchner analyze the relationships between the social and professional characteristics of physicians and their attitudes toward social issues. Social and professional characteristics are conceptualized as "social statuses (defined as positions in a social system [Merton 1957: 368]), and as sources of socialization" (1986: 74). Social statuses such as gender and race/ethnicity condition the social experiences of individuals in patterned ways, so that we see, for example, differential patterns of medical specialization and practice setting by gender and race/ethnicity. Women, for example, have traditionally been overrepresented in the medical specialty of pediatrics and in institutional practice settings (Bowman and Gross 1986: 516). African Americans are overrepresented in the primary care specialties (USDHHS 1993: 11) and underrepresented in group practice settings (USDHHS 1993: 14).

In turn, professional statuses such as specialty and practice setting may influence physicians' experiences, attitudes, and behavior. Psychiatrists, for example, are more likely to have more liberal attitudes than other physicians, and solo practitioners are more likely to hold more conservative attitudes about the role of government in medicine than physicians in other types of practices. Colombotos and Kirchner emphasize, however, that social selection may also explain differences in physicians' attitudes. Psychiatry may draw a subgroup of physicians with more liberal attitudes into its ranks. They also emphasize that experiences and situations are "continuous sources of socialization" (1986: 76) and that, in addition to the experiences acquired during formal training and education, later work experiences may influence attitudes of individuals in important ways (1986: 75).

Relationships Among Statuses, Attitudes, and Ideology

Professional ideology may be conceptualized as a set of attitudes governing the work of a prestigious occupation. Colombotos (1969) has examined the relationship between physician background characteristics and attitudes toward professional values such as service and commitment versus economic rewards and prestige.

Another aspect of the professional ideology of physicians may be conceptualized as a set of professional norms related to ethical obligation to treat and legal obligations toward patients. The manner in which physicians of different social origins and professional characteristics respond to the norms regarding ethical and legal obligation may vary. In general, female, minority, and foreign-educated physicians have been found to be more politically liberal than their respective colleagues (Colombotos 1969; Colombotos, Charles, and Kirchner 1977; Richard 1969; Colombotos and Kirchner 1986). Colombotos et al. (1995) found that liberal political ideology of health care workers is positively related to their professional obligation to treat patients with HIV.

SUMMARY OF HYPOTHESES

In summary, prior research supports the plausibility of the following relationships to explain physician participation in Medicaid: social statuses (gender, race/ethnicity, foreign birthplace) influence physicians' participation in Medicaid both directly and indirectly through their professional statuses and characteristics and ideology. Professional statuses (international medical graduate, no board certification, specialty) and practice characteristics (institutional setting, low-income location) influence physicians' participation in Medicaid directly and indirectly through ideology. Physicians' political and professional ideologies influence their participation in Medicaid directly.

CAUSAL MODEL

The relationships among social status, professional status and characteristics, political and professional ideology, and Medicaid participation may be depicted within a framework of marginality. *Social marginality* (defined on the basis of female gender, minority race/ethnicity, or foreign birthplace status) leads to *professional marginality* (foreign medical school, no board certification, specialty choice, institutional practice setting, practice location with a high minority population, practice location with a high poverty population). Both social and professional marginality are expected to influence *physician ideology*. Social marginality and professional marginality are expected to directly and indirectly influence physician participation in Medicaid while ideology is expected to directly influence physician participation in Medicaid. Figure 2.1 depicts these relationships.

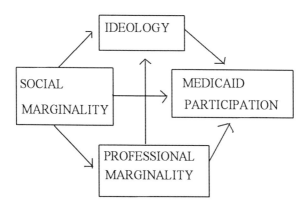

Figure 2.1 Causal Model of Medicaid Participation

While acknowledging the important role of social and professional statuses in determining a series of career choices and professional attitudes of physicians, this study posits that the social experience of marginality dominates the socialization of certain groups within the medical profession. In other words, the social experience of being female, minority, or foreign-born and foreign-educated dominates an individual's socialization within the medical profession and consequently influences the individual's political and professional ideology. Marginal statuses are cumulative; that is, more marginal social statuses lead to the accumulation of more marginal professional statuses.

DEFINITION OF MARGINALITY AND MARGINALIZATION

Marginality is a social condition associated with long-standing social and economic barriers and may be the end result of a process of formal and/or informal discrimination. Classic examples of marginality involve those groups who are historically recognized as having been discriminated against in the larger society. I use the term "marginalization" to characterize either an intentional or unintentional process whereby particular social statuses are considered less desirable for positions within an institution or profession. Individuals possessing "inappropriate" statuses are, for the most part, relegated to the "margins" in less desirable positions of the profession. The process is cumulative, so that the person of less valued social status is viewed as less deserving and, consequently given fewer opportunities, resulting in an "accumulation of marginality." Marginalization, while not outright segregation, falls short of full professional integration.

CONCLUSION

More than two decades of empirical studies of office-based physicians suggest that economic self-interest and physician shortages in low-income areas are factors associated with physician participation in Medicaid. In view of trends away from office-based primary care for Medicaid patients, it is worthwhile to look at physicians in different practice settings with respect to their participation in Medicaid.

Chapter Three elaborates a theoretical framework that explains how ascribed social statuses (female gender, minority race/ethnicity, and foreign birthplace) are likely to lead to professionally marginal statuses and thereby influence those physicians' participation in Medicaid. This framework offers a conceptual guide for the empirical findings of this study.

It should be emphasized that this study is not rejecting the economic model but rather complementing it with social theory. The assumption implicit in the economic two-market theory—a behavioral one of self-interest—may be augmented by inclusion of social status variables such as gender, race/ethnicity, U.S. or foreign birthplace, as well as ideological variables. The addition of these variables is helpful in that they elucidate the social processes at work that result in social stratification within the U.S. medical profession which, consequently, influences who cares for poor Medicaid patients. As a result, we have a more complete explanation for the social phenomenon. The marginalization and socialization frameworks help us conceptualize the social processes associated with physicians' participation in Medicaid.

Since this study consists of a secondary analysis of cross-sectional data, it does not permit a thorough investigation of all the social processes described in the theoretical framework; however, I believe that an understanding of the social processes elaborated in this study may add to understanding of physician participation in Medicaid and guide future investigations.

NOTES

1. In 1990, the American Medical Association began using the term "International Medical Graduate" or "IMG" to refer to physicians trained in medical schools outside of the U.S. Previous to this time, such physicians were referred to as "Foreign Medical Graduates" or "FMGs." In this book, I use the terms International Medical Graduate and IMG except when quoting research conducted prior to 1990.

2. Sloan et al. (1978) asked physicians if they agreed or disagreed with this statement: "There are too many controls on the medical profession that interfere with taking care of patients" (1978: 121).

3. Specifically, Perloff et al. (1987a) ask the following question: "Some people believe it is the responsibility of society, through its government, to ensure that medical care is available to those who cannot afford it. Do you: agree with that strongly, agree somewhat, disagree somewhat or disagree strongly?" Sloan et al. (1978: 121) ask a similarly worded question.

III

Marginality in the Medical Profession

CONCEPTUAL ISSUES

Background

The historic underrepresentation of women and minorities in the U.S. medical profession has been well documented (USDHHS 1990a; USDHHS 1993). Underrepresentation in medicine is a product of long-term social barriers, outright exclusion, and quotas for women and particularly African Americans, the largest minority group in the U.S. (Walsh 1977; Morantz-Sanchez 1985; Shea and Fullilove 1985; Taylor, Hunt, and Temple 1990; Petersdorf 1992). In recent years, policymakers and advocates within the profession have argued for an increase in the number of women and minorities in the belief that these groups of physicians will be more likely to provide primary care to urban minority and other medically underserved populations (USDHHS 1990a, 1990b; USDHHS 1993; Rivo and Satcher 1993; Steinbrook 1996).

Empirical investigations indicate that women and minority physicians do indeed treat larger numbers of poor and minority patients (Adams and Bazzoli 1986; Hojat et al. 1990; USDHHS 1993; Komaromy et al. 1996; Cantor et al. 1996). According to a 1987 American Medical Association (AMA) survey of young physicians, blacks comprise approximately 50 percent of the patient load of young black physicians compared to about ten percent of that of all other physicians; Hispanics comprise about 20 percent of the patient load of young Hispanic physicians compared to about five percent of that of all other physicians. Young black physicians are more likely than other racial/ethnic groups to serve low-income patients (Keith et al. 1985; USDHHS 1993: iii).[1]

Hojat et al's (1990) study of graduates from Jefferson Medical College between 1977 and 1981 found that female physicians were significantly more likely than male physicians to treat low-income patients and to work in underserved areas in large cities. They conclude: "If these trends are general ones, women physicians may increasingly fill important gaps in the medical profession and may contribute to the solution of the physician maldistribution problem" (Hojat et al. 1990).

In their analysis of data from the AMA's 1983 national Survey of Resident Physicians, Adams and Bazzoli (1986) note that women were significantly more likely than men to choose primary care specialties and that, of the four racial/ethnic-gender groupings, minority women were most likely to choose primary care specialties. Thirty-five percent of white men, 45 percent of minority men, 47 percent of white women, and 70 percent of minority women planned to practice primary care.[2] Adams and Bazzoli also found that minority resident physicians were significantly more likely than all other residents to plan to practice in urban areas (Adams and Bazzoli 1986: 20).

Komaromy et al. (1996) analyzed California physicians' practice locations and the racial/ethnic composition and socioeconomic status of those communities in 1990. In 1993, they also surveyed primary care physicians in California regarding their race/ethnicity and the characteristics of their patient population. They found that communities with high percentages of black and Hispanics were significantly more likely to experience a physician shortage, even after controlling for income levels of those communities. They also found that black physicians cared for significantly more black patients, while Hispanic physicians cared for significantly more Hispanic patients compared to all other physicians. In addition, black physicians were significantly more likely to care for Medicaid patients and Hispanic physicians were significantly more likely to care for more uninsured patients than all other physicians.

Cantor et al. (1996) used data from the 1987 and 1991 Surveys of Young Physicians, two large-scale surveys of physicians age 40-or-under at first interview and in practice for at least one year, to examine the social status of physicians and their patient populations. They found that female and minority physicians were significantly more likely than white male physicians, to serve poor, minority, and Medicaid patients. Black and Hispanic female physicians provided the most care to poor and Medicaid patients. White female and minority male physicians provided more care to these patient populations compared to white male physicians but to a lesser extent than black and Hispanic female physicians. Cantor et al. also found that physicians who expressed a high motivation to care for specific minority groups or to those patients having trouble obtaining care did, in fact, provide care to significantly greater proportions of these patients compared to physicians expressing low motivation.

An extensive literature supports the notion that social factors affect physicians' choice of specialty (Kandel 1960; Kritzer and Zimet 1967; Weisman et al. 1980; Harris and Conley-Muth 1981; Schermerhorn et al. 1986; Nager and Saadatmand 1991), type of practice (Westling-Wikstrand, Monk, and Thomas 1970), hospital appointments (Solomon 1961), academic appointments (Westling-Wikstrand, Monk, and Thomas 1970; Rinke 1981a), and patient clientele (Lieberson 1958; Hojat et al. 1990; Adams and Bazzoli 1986; Komaromy et al. 1996; Cantor et al. 1996). Bergner's study of New Jersey physicians (1970) found that their social backgrounds influenced their medical career paths from at least the start of medical school. Bergner notes that "the dependence works in two ways. It may influence the student or trainee or hospital appointee to seek positions only at particular institutions or locations. And it may indicate an institution's preference for students or physicians with certain characteristics" (Bergner 1970: 245). The social patterning of specialty, practice type, and practice location in the medical profession is of continuing interest to policymakers and researchers today (USDHHS 1990, 1993; Komaromy et al. 1996; Cantor et al. 1996; Mick and Lee 1997).

Although government policy analysts underscore the national need for more primary care physicians, primary care medical practice remains a less desirable and prestigious alternative within the U.S. medical profession (USDHHS 1990b). In a study of African American physicians in New York City, Richard (1969) observed that an important indicator of professional integration, or acceptance within the profession, is the percentage of specialists in the minority group. Specialized practice typically requires at least three years of advanced training, is more lucrative, and is thereby considered more prestigious than general practice (Stern 1958). The facts that female and minority physicians are much less likely than male and white physicians to specialize, and when specializing are more likely to choose the lower-paying primary care specialties (Altekruse and McDermott 1988; Babbott, Weaver, and Baldwin 1994) are strong indications that they have not achieved full integration within the medical profession.

Among the medical specialties, pediatrics has the highest proportion of female to male physicians (Langwell 1982; Bowman and Gross 1986; AMA 1992) and is also the lowest paying medical specialty, with a per hourly rate of income lower even than that of general practice (Bobula 1980). Given the fact that children under the age of 18 comprise the highest proportion of low-income Americans, it is quite likely that pediatricians also treat higher proportions of low-income Americans than do other specialist types.

Adams and Bazzoli also observe that women are overrepresented in salaried hospital-based positions and Health Maintenance Organizations (HMOs) and suggest that such patterns are not simply a reflection of gender differences in risk-taking. They argue that, since the same pattern of difference exists between minority and white physicians (minorities are also overrepresented in salaried hospital-based positions and HMOs), "additional factors must be at work...Anticipated patient or peer discrimination may make (office-based) practice undesirable...In addition, minority physicians may perceive barriers to entry into (private) group practices due to the dominance of white physicians in most groups" (Adams and Bazzoli 1986: 20). Adams and Bazzoli's findings, which are supported by data from the American Medical Association (AMA 1991, 1992; UDHHS 1993), show that "distinctive patterns in career choice" exist among race/ethnicity and gender groupings.

This chapter draws on social theory to explore whether and how the marginalization of certain social status social groupings (female, minority, foreign-born and foreign-educated) in society is linked to their marginalization in the medical profession. Before exploring marginality in the medical profession, I will first trace the origins of the concept.

The Marginal Man Concept

Notions of "the marginal man" are legendary throughout the literary, scientific, and sociological worlds.[3] The concept has been widely used by some (Park 1928; Stonequist 1961; Hughes 1971; Willie 1975) and sharply criticized by others (Golovensky 1952; Gieryn and Hirsh 1983).[4]

The concept of the marginal man was first formulated by the sociologist Robert E. Park and later elaborated upon by his student of the Chicago school, Everett V. Stonequist. It describes an individual who, shaped by one culture and later brought into permanent contact with another culture, finds him or herself on the periphery of both cultures, but truly belonging to neither. Park's classic example of the marginal man is the Jewish immigrant in America, the person who emerges from the European ghetto "seeking to find a place in the freer, more complex and cosmopolitan life of an American city" (Park 1928: 892). Park describes him as:

> a cultural hybrid, a man living and sharing intimately in
> the cultural life and traditions of two distinct peoples;
> never quite willing to break, even if he were permitted to
> do so, with his past and his traditions, and not quite
> accepted, because of racial prejudice, in the new society
> in which he now sought to find a place. He was a man on
> the margin of two cultures and two societies which never
> completely interpenetrated and fused (1928: 892).

Park notes that the marginal man's conception of himself is constructed by the opinions and attitudes of other persons in his society. The individual falls prey to a type of dual personality resulting from this socially determined position. Stonequist observes:

> One sees this social dislocation clearly and sharply in the
> case of those individuals who fall between two major
> racial or cultural groups...the individual who through
> migration, education, marriage, or some other influence
> leaves one social group or culture without making a
> satisfactory adjustment to another finds himself on the
> margin of each but a member of neither (1961:2-3).

Stonequist acknowledges that the changes in the traditional role of
women produces similar "dilemmas in ambition and conduct." He notes
that, as work within the home declines and opportunities outside the home
increase, women's movement into the workforce and professions tends to
result in a backlash of public sentiment and morals: "The pioneers thus
find themselves between two fires: men who resist their encroachment,
and women who are outraged by their free and seemingly adventurous
conduct" (1961: 8). The consequence of ostracization for the marginal
person is exclusion from "numerous spheres of social activity—from a
system of group relationships" (1961: 7-8). The marginal person functions
on the periphery of group life.

It is from the standpoint of status that Everett C. Hughes (1971)
examines the phenomenon of marginality. In his view, status is a socially
ascribed or achieved position embedded within a particular culture, with
attendant rights, limitations, and duties and acted out within "a system of
relations between people." This notion of status approximates Merton's
definition of status as a "position in a social system occupied by designated
individuals" and role as "the behavioral enacting of the patterned
expectations attributed to that position." Merton describes status and role
as "concepts connecting the culturally defined expectations with the
patterned behavior and relationships which comprise social structure"
(Merton, 1957: 368).

Hughes, like Park and Stonequist, discusses the marginal man both
from an internal, psychological and external, sociological perspective. In
my discussion of marginality within the medical profession, I refer

specifically to the external manifestations of marginalization in the profession. Certainly, there are profound psychological consequences of marginalization that impact upon an individual's career choices; nevertheless, it is beyond the scope of this book to analyze this aspect of the phenomenon.

Hughes elaborates upon the notion of marginal man as "a man with a status dilemma," noting that, as an individual acquires elements of culture that accord success and higher position to others, the greater is that person's dilemma (1971: 220). Marginality occurs "wherever there is sufficient social change going on to allow the emergence of people who are in a position of confusion of social identity, with its attendant conflicts of loyalty and frustration of personal and group aspirations" (1971: 225-226). A prime example, he observes, is the African American person who historically has been assigned a "limited" social status but who may possess other characteristics (such as a highly regarded profession) that would ordinarily assign to him or her a higher status. Using the example of a black physician, Hughes notes that this phenomenon presents a social contradiction that is an apparent contradiction to the social world in which the person lives.

Certain statuses are dominant over others in most societies. Epstein (1971) notes that:

> Certain ascribed statuses—sex status and racial status, for example—are central in controlling the choices of most individuals. The status of 'woman' is one such dominant and often salient status. For a woman, sex status is primary and pivotal and it inevitably determines much of the course of her life, especially because of rigid cultural definitions which limit the range of other statuses she may acquire (1971: 92).

Epstein's argument is consistent with Colombotos and Kirchner's observation that "longer and more stable" sources of socialization, such as gender and ethnicity, may exert a greater effect than more recently acquired statuses on personal attitudes (1986: 81).

Marginality in the Professions

Certain social positions possess a "a halo of technically irrelevant, but socially expected characteristics" (Hughes 1971: 222-223). This phenomenon, discussed at length by sociologists (Merton 1957: 370; Epstein 1971: 87; Lorber 1984) is one that Epstein (1971) characterizes as "status-set typing," noting that it "occurs when a class of persons shares statuses *and when it is considered appropriate that they do so*" (Epstein 1971: 87). The upper echelons of many professions are "status-set typed" in the sense that members expect and prefer that individuals possess not only the status relevant to their profession, but also other statuses irrelevant to their professional performance. A prime example is the neurosurgeon, a high status medical specialist (Schwartzbaum and McGrath 1973; Shortell 1974) who commonly holds other statuses such as male gender and white race. These additional statuses appear to "complement" the occupational status. An atypical combination of statuses within one individual, an African American female neurosurgeon, for example, tends to create discomfort among colleague group members. Status-sets which appear particularly natural effectively limit other combinations. Epstein notes that "to the extent that a status is institutionalized within a body of other statuses the range of other possible combinations of statuses will be limited" (1971: 92).

In professions, the colleague group acts in subtle but powerful ways to create very specific expectations regarding auxiliary statuses its members should possess (Etzioni 1961; Epstein 1971: 167). These auxiliary statuses become, as Hughes notes, a basis for the colleague group's definition of its common interests and formal code and how it selects those who become part of the inner circle:

> In order that men may communicate freely and confidentially, they must be able to take a good deal of each other's sentiments for granted. They must feel easy about their silences as well as about their utterances. These factors conspire to make colleagues, with a large body of unspoken understandings, uncomfortable in the

> presence of what they consider odd kinds of fellows. The
> person who is the first of his kind to attain a certain status
> is often not drawn into the informal brotherhood in which
> experiences are exchanged, competence built up, and the
> formal code elaborated and enforced. He thus remains
> forever a marginal man (Hughes 1971: 146).

Who exactly constitutes this group of "odd kinds of fellows" differs across historical periods, cultures, and types of colleague groups. The medical profession in the United States has historically been male-dominated, and at various periods has effectively relegated "unwanted," "inappropriate" groups (such as immigrants, Catholics, Jews, African Americans, women) to the periphery of the profession or, in some cases, has limited their numbers deliberately (Lopate 1968; Walsh 1977; Starr 1982).

Exclusion from the various spheres of professional life typically takes place through formal or informal barriers to advancement. Sponsorship, an informal mechanism, is widely practiced in the medical profession as a means of advancing careers of young physicians. It is simultaneously a powerful barrier to advancement of other young physicians' careers. Sponsorship, then, can be viewed as a dual mechanism involving the promotion of some and the "boycott" of others (Lorber 1984: 6; Freidson 1970: 185-201). A dominant status group may avoid overt exclusion of undesirable status groups through the use of mechanisms like sponsorship and boycott. The informality of these mechanisms makes them particularly powerful.

The Role of Sponsorship

Sponsorship is the central facet of a social process of career building. In his classic study of physicians in a small community in the 1940s, Oswald Hall documented the manner in which physicians organized themselves into homogenous groups. A dominant core of specialist practitioners exerted control through hospital appointments and posts, a less powerful "friendly" group were dependent upon them for referrals, and an outer group of isolated "individualists" operated independently (Hall 1946, 1948, 1949). The inner elite sponsored novice physicians who possessed the appropriate demeanor and social characteristics through a series of resources and rewards, most notably referrals, hospital privileges, partnerships, staff appointments, and organizational memberships. In this way, the favored novices were groomed to become members of the powerful and prestigious inner circle; simultaneously, the less favored were relegated to peripheral positions in the medical community. Hall observed that sponsorship is the primary means by which medical careers progress:

> By sponsorship is meant simply that established members of the inner fraternity actively intervene in the career lines of newcomers to the profession. By so doing they influence the careers of those selected...Sponsorship has a dual purpose. It facilitates the careers of those selected and relegates those not so selected to a position where they compete under decidedly disadvantageous terms (Hall 1946: 32-33).

He identified the channels through which younger doctors of the appropriate class and ethnic origins were absorbed into an inner circle of the medical profession as well as the ways in which persons whose status-sets were deemed inappropriate were excluded from the system. He noted that the practice of medicine "is carried on within the framework of elaborate social machinery" (1946: 336) and that a key facet of a successful medical career "involves acceptance by the inner fraternity" (1946: 335-356).

More recently, A.E. Miller (1977) has argued that although the locus of professional power has shifted away from the small community office-based physicians, the sponsor-protégé relationship is still the pattern for advancement in the medical profession. In a longitudinal survey of a national sample of physicians graduated from medical school in 1960, Marshall, Fulton, and Wessen (1978) examined the process of medical education and career outcomes. They found that the formal system of medical education is complemented by an informal system centered on the sponsor-protégé relationship and concluded that:

> Sponsorship may be seen as a means of subverting the more egalitarian formal system. Instead of letting those who can rise to the top do so, sponsorship seems to accelerate the rise of some while suppressing the chances of others. Most importantly, it is not clear from our data what criteria are being used to select who moves up, who moves down, and who gets a chance to compete (Marshall et al. 1978: 135).

Each stage of medical education (premedical, medical, graduate, postgraduate, and eventual practice) is part of a continuous process comprised of formal and informal processes (Marshall et al. 1978). The formal system (which includes college grade point average, the medical school admissions test [MCAT], frequent tests, a structured curriculum, national exams, and faculty evaluations) reinforces the belief that individual motivation and achievement determine success. Numerous studies, however, have documented a parallel informal system that functions "to sort out students based upon individual statuses and guide them into the prestige hierarchy of professional medicine" (Marshall et al. 1978: 125; see also Hall 1949; Back et al. 1958; Krause 1971).

The Social Process of Career Building

There are several mechanisms identified by theorists and researchers (Goode 1957; Epstein 1970, 1971; Kanter 1977; Reskin 1978; Mumford 1970; Lorber 1984) that describe the "sorting and sifting" processes of career building. The sociological notion of "status expectations" posits that ascribed statuses like female gender, foreign birth, and minority race/ethnicity, powerfully influence

social interaction by limiting the opportunities for

performance, particularly in positions of authority, of
those of devalued status. Those of higher status are
assumed to be competent and are automatically accepted
for leadership roles; those of lower status have the burden
of proof—they must establish their competence and their
legitimacy as potential leaders (Lorber 1984: 4-5).

Through a series of processes stemming from status expectations,
persons of devalued social status are relegated to peripheral positions
within the social structure. Lorber argues that status expectations are one
manifestation of the "Matthew effect," the process described by Merton
(1968) and Zuckerman (1977) whereby Nobel scientists accumulate
social advantages and visibility.[5] Lorber notes that the accumulation of
advantages by "the haves" is essentially an invisible process, in that
"those in positions of power, authority, privilege, and wealth, as well as
those doubly deprived, usually accept the inequities as legitimate" (1984:
5). Achievement-oriented societies, such as the United States, operate on
a common assumption that if you work hard, you can get ahead, so it is
expected that the talented, motivated person can transcend the limits of
class, gender, and ethnicity to compete on a level playing field with
universalistic criteria.

The fairness of the Matthew effect has been debated in academic
circles (Cole 1979; Martin 1982; Tuchman 1980). Lorber argues that it is
highly debatable whether competition for the prestige positions in
professional hierarchies is open and whether achievement based on
objective standards applied equally to all is the primary evaluative
criterion. She, like Hall and Hughes, argues that the dominant members of
professional groups set the standards, control the opportunities, and
attempt to maintain their values and ideas by selecting protégés like
themselves.

The sponsored novice is given opportunities to demonstrate
competency and gain visibility within the larger professional group.

Lorber notes:

> If protégés were chosen by sponsors strictly on the basis
> of their potential, as demonstrated by their performance
> during training, the system would be based on merit.
> However, the choice of colleagues and successors is also
> usually made on the basis of other criteria, such as race
> and gender (1984: 6).

Overt discrimination is no longer legally or socially tolerated, but rejection on the basis of technically irrelevant statuses does occur. Lorber informs us that evaluation based on social characteristics of the protégé is not a conspiracy, nor is it confined to the medical profession. Rather, "it is a pervasive and persistent social phenomenon that can be found in every profession and occupation" (1984: 7).

Lorber identifies another process that limits the career mobility of individuals who possess inappropriate status-sets in professions. The "Salieri phenomenon," refers to the court composer Salieri who posed as a benefactor to the young Mozart but who, in fact, blocked opportunities for his advancement. It describes the subtle denigration of an individual's professional worth within larger colleague networks: "This process is often invisible to the recipients and frequently unconscious on the part of the perpetrators, particularly when merit and performance are supposed to be the prevailing evaluative criteria" (1984: 9). She adds that the Salieri phenomenon is not indiscriminately used against all newcomers with unacceptable traits or social backgrounds; rather it is used selectively against those who, questioning the prevailing values and beliefs, might establish new standards. Individuals who dominate the colleague circles tend to judge the performance and behavior of newcomers by the standards and values of the social group to which they belong rather than by objective or universalistic standards (1984: 10).

Colleague groups are oftentimes based on common auxiliary statuses such as gender, race, or ethnicity (Lorber 1984: 5). The phenomenon of "invisible colleges," communities of professionals who have trained together and hold consensus on the quality of work, is pervasive in academic medical centers and research settings (Lorber 1984; Cole, Cole, and Simon 1981; Latour and Woolgar 1979; Crane 1972; Miller 1970). The practice of medicine is controlled by peer regulation, and the dual mechanisms of sponsorship and boycott function to produce professional networks that are homogeneous with respect to certain qualities and standards of performance (Freidson 1970: 185-201; Lorber 1984: 6).

In the following sections, I will examine the empirical literature describing the career patterns of women, minority, and foreign-born and foreign-educated physicians in the United States.

WOMEN IN MEDICINE

Career Patterns of Women Physicians

Formal and informal institutional barriers excluded women from U.S. medical schools up until 1970 (Heins 1985). In her study of women in the professions, Epstein (1970) observed that both women and racial minorities find that the institutionalized channels of recruitment and advancement are not available to them because their sexual or racial status within the professions is seen as inappropriate. The medical profession in the United States has undergone vast changes since 1970; nevertheless, Epstein's observation is relevant to the racial and sexual division of labor we see in the medical profession today. The number of women in the medical profession has increased dramatically in recent years. Between the years 1970 and 1990 the number of female physicians in the United States nearly quadrupled. In 1992, 18 percent of all physicians and 42 percent of medical students were women. By the year 2010, women are expected to comprise 30 percent of the physician workforce (Bickel and Kopriva 1993: 41). The apparent gains by women, however, are undercut by the concentration of women in the less prestigious, lower paying specialties and positions in the medical profession.

Once medical school training is completed, career paths of male and female physicians are strikingly dissimilar. Women enter the primary care specialties at a higher rate. They are also overrepresented in institutional settings with fixed, regular work hours. About 70 percent of female physicians practice in internal medicine, pediatrics, family practice, and psychiatry. These are the lowest paid specialties (Nadelson 1991: 95).

One explanation for gendered patterns of specialty choice is that both informal and formal barriers effectively block women from entering more prestigious specialties that have historically been exclusive male domains. The sponsor-protégé system in the medical profession is an informal but highly effective way to prevent certain groups from entering particular specialties.

In her study of specialty choice among male and female physicians in training, Davidson (1979) examined two other commonly cited reasons for female physicians' distinctive career patterns—sex role compatibility and time demands. Sex role compatibility has been offered most commonly as the explanation for the concentration of women in pediatrics, psychiatry, and public health (Kosa and Coker 1965). This argument states that certain specialties are more compatible with traditional female roles than others, specifically those that require empathy and nurturance; in order to avoid role conflict, female physicians tend to choose specialties that are more compatible with other roles (i.e., wife and mother) they play. One could argue, however, that other traditionally male specialties such as ophthalmology, which offer regular hours and require a "delicate touch," are also better suited to the traditional female role; yet, women are underrepresented in such high prestige specialties. The role compatibility argument reinforces rigid sex role definitions of specialties and, as Davidson points out, it reminds women that:

> there are a *few* places in medicine for them, but not too *many*...to the extent that women choose medical specialties because those specialties are task compatible with traditional sex role stereotypes, that choice is a 'choice by constraint' (1979: 201-203).

Cross-national studies point out the diverse way in which professions are gender-typed and, as such, indicate that popular beliefs about the appropriateness of certain fields or subfields for women are simply ex-post facto rationalizations for the gendered division of labor. Whereas in the

United States medicine has traditionally been viewed as a detached, scientifically oriented profession, it has been defined as an expressive, nurturant profession well-suited for women in the Soviet Union (Epstein 1971: 151-166).

Another explanation for the concentration of women in particular specialties and practice settings relates to time demands (Kosa and Coker 1965). Women choose those specialties and practice settings that provide regular hours, thereby reducing the role conflicts arising between professional obligations and traditional sex role obligations to family and home. It is worth noting that this conflict involves time, not necessarily any "intrinsic functional incompatibility" between a female's practice and gender. Davidson observes:

> One might argue that the task compatibility and time constraints are partially self-imposed and based on internal motivation. Yet internal motivation must be viewed as a product of long standing external imposition of traditional female role definitions and status obligations. Clearly, denial of access to or discouragement from entering any specialty is an external constraint, whether that denial is based on institutional policy or informal pressure exerted by individual members within a conventional structure (1979: 203).

Davidson (1979) found, in her sample of physicians in training, that both sex role compatibility and time demand issues "interact to constrain women's selection of specialty." She noted that, in contrast to male physicians, females' specialty choices appeared to be "expedient adjustments aimed at maximizing role compatibility and minimizing conflict between two statuses rather than at fulfilling the physician's preferred professional interest" (1979: 213). Women physicians-in-training, in contrast to the men, felt obligated to pick specialties in their interest area with the greatest number of institutional positions followed by a subspecialty offering fixed working hours. Davidson concludes that women physicians' choice of specialty reflects their conscious attempts to minimize role conflicts. Women physicians in her study recognized that the medical profession offered a limited number of positions for women as well as a limited choice of specialties (1979: 213-214).

Davidson disputes the usefulness of professional norms, noting that traditional advice for women to train for particular specialties is simply to advise women to adjust to the existing limitations within particular specialties, rather than question the functional utility of the way in which work is structured:

> To track women into scheduled specialties, regardless of the substantive content of those specialties, is a token, not a structural solution to a real problem. It is an attempt to fit a task to available time rather than to fit time for a wide and open range of available tasks. Such an approach is neither sensible nor functional for effective medical care (1979: 215).

Career Development of Women Physicians

Additional insights into the career development of female and male physicians is provided by Lorber and Ecker's (1983) research. Using a matched sample of female and male physicians who graduated from medical school in 1960 and were followed through 1976, Lorber and Ecker analyzed the effects of several variables commonly associated with professional attainment: achievement motivation, performance in medical school, peer evaluation, prestige of internship hospital, and family responsibilities. They found that only a very small proportion of the variance in professional attainment, for men (13 percent) as well as women (14 percent), is explained by the factors studied, observing that "much of the important informal aspect of career advancement is missing from these models, particularly the help that established physicians extend to novices in hospital appointments, practice arrangement, referrals, and consultations" (Lorber and Ecker 1983: 454).

The variables Lorber and Ecker studied were those commonly attributed to account for differences among male and female physicians' professional achievements. The authors found that achievement motivation and performance in medical school were stronger predictors of professional attainment for men than for women. Prestige of internship hospital, although statistically significant for both men and women, was a particularly strong predictor for women. Family responsibility had negative effects for females' but not males' professional attainment (Lorber and Ecker 1983).

In comparing males' and females' professional attainment after 16 years, the authors found that male physicians had significantly higher professional attainment than female physicians. The various factors examined by the study appeared to assist men's careers in a sustained, chronological manner, while fewer factors were associated with professional attainment among women. Path analytic models indicated that men with high achievement motivation tended to have high national exam scores, high peer and faculty evaluations, high junior year standings, and high-prestige internships (Lorber and Ecker 1983).

Among women, high national exam scores and high prestige internship were unrelated to each other but were independently strong predictors of high professional attainment. Achievement motivation was associated with high peer evaluations; however, peer evaluations were not associated with any other independent variables or with professional attainment. Faculty evaluations were not associated with high professional attainment for women. Family responsibilities did not have direct effects on males', but did have negative direct effects on females', attainments. Lorber observes:

> Given this cross-cutting of factors in their careers, women physicians may have increased their family responsibilities because of the limits on their professional attainment, rather than limiting their professional commitments because of increased family responsibilities, as is usually thought (1984: 46-47).

Lorber and Ecker's analysis underscores the fact that traits commonly thought to predict career success of male and female physicians actually explain very little of the variation in achievement, suggesting that other factors such as sponsorship may provide important links to career success.

The importance of the mentoring relationship in medicine for training and career advancement has been echoed by advocates within the profession (Sirridge 1985; Petersdorf 1990; Lenhart 1993; DeAngelis 1995). Lenhart observes that key decisionmakers within the hierarchy of medicine control a variety of professional opportunities for new entrants and "potential mentors who are unaccustomed to or uncomfortable with relating to women as colleagues or who still perceive women as subordinates and caretakers will exclude women or limit their access to mentors" (1993: 155-56). Sirridge offers suggestions for protégés, noting that mentors provide valuable assistance in increasing their visibility and opportunities for further training and research. In 1990, the president of the Association of American Medical Colleges, Robert Petersdorf, called for more research in the area of mentoring in medical education. In a 1988 survey of faculty members at the Medical College of Wisconsin, Kirsling and Kochar (1990) found that among those faculty who reported having had a mentor, the vast majority agreed that the relationship had assisted their personal development, helped them cope with stress, and promoted their career development.

Changing Proportions of Women in Medicine

It should be emphasized that marginality is not a static condition. As population dynamics shift or assimilation occurs, one status group may be absorbed into the mainstream, while another status group may emerge as marginal. The recent dramatic increase in the number of women in the medical profession raises the question as to whether women are still marginal in the medical profession of 1998.

In a classic study of American corporate life, Kanter (1993) argues that the proportions ("the social composition of people in approximately the same situation") in which a group finds itself determines its social experience in an organization. Those who hold a minority, and consequently, marginal status within a work group typically face "the loneliness of the stranger who intrudes upon an alien culture." Kanter argues that it is scarcity rather than inherent "otherness" that creates marginality. As groups become balanced proportionately, organizational culture and interaction change to reflect this balance and individuals' opportunities and experience depend less on their marginal status and more on other structural and personal factors (Kanter 1993: 207-209).

Although other researchers agree with Kanter that the skewed proportions of minority groups in the workplace contribute to the problem of marginalization, they also argue that increasing numbers alone will not alleviate problems once marginal people occupy positions as peers (Buono and Kamm 1983: 1129; Lorber 1984: 111). Lorber points to the "glass ceiling" phenomenon whereby women are denied access to top positions by a combination of sexism built into the structure of career mobility as well as deep seated sexism of elite men (Reskin 1988; Lorber 1993: 64). The glass ceiling has been identified in every male-dominated profession which women have entered in the last two decades (Blum and Smith 1988; Lorber 1993). The difficulty women have in integrating themselves into high prestige positions and the illusion that women have fully incorporated themselves within the medical profession is illustrated by the case of women in medical academia.

Women in Medical Academia

Researchers and advocates within the medical profession have noted the differentials in rank and promotion between men and women in medical academia (Bickel and Kopriva 1993; DeAngelis and Johns 1995; Tesch et al. 1995; Kirschstein 1996). Using data drawn from the Association of American Medical Colleges (AAMC) and the AMA, Bickel and Kopriva (1993) found that since 1970, the proportion of female faculty in medical schools has grown steadily. Between 1970 and 1992, the number of women faculty grew 130 percent compared to 52 percent for men. Approximately 22 percent of full-time medical school faculty members were women in 1992 compared to less than 16 percent in 1980. In fact, about 14 percent of female compared to ten percent of male medical school graduates become full-time faculty members. This phenomenon is most likely due to females' greater tendency to seek salaried positions compared to their male counterparts (Bickel and

Kopriva 1993: 142).

Within medical faculties, however, great discrepancies are seen in terms of rank. Male faculty are more evenly spread over the three ranks of full professor, associate professor, and assistant professor whereas the majority of women are assistant professors.[6] While critics may argue that these discrepancies are simply a function of age and experience (women tend to be younger), among the cohort who first became faculty in 1976, only ten percent of the women compared to 22 percent of the men had reached the rank of professor by 1991 (Bickel and Kopriva: 143).

Twenty percent of all male faculty were tenured in 1992 compared to five percent of all female faculty. Males comprised 93 percent of all tenured professors. Among non-tenure-track faculty, the proportion of women increased with decreasing rank, so that they comprised 41 percent of all non-tenure-track instructors.

In recent years, approximately 75 percent of U.S. medical schools have created a clinician-educator track as a promotion ladder for clinical teaching faculty. Bickel and Kopriva examined 13 schools with separate tenure and clinician-educator tracks and found that 18 percent of the male faculty, in contrast to 26 percent of the female faculty, had appointments as clinician-educators, lending credibility to the impression that women are concentrated in less prestigious tracks (Bickel and Kopriva 1993).

Bickel and Kopriva's findings are consistent with those of Tesch et al. (1995) who, in 1992, surveyed a sample of male and female physician faculty in U.S. medical schools. Both groups of physicians, first appointed between 1979 and 1981, were asked questions regarding their academic rank, academic productivity, academic resources, career preparedness and family responsibilities. They found that while 83 percent of the men had become associate or full professor only 59 percent of the women had, and 23 percent of the men compared to five percent of the women were full professors after an average of 11 years on a medical school faculty. Tesch and colleagues found that women were significantly less likely to achieve associate or full professor rank compared to men and that this was not explained by controlling for academic productivity factors.

Faculty's perceptions of their work environments also lend some insights into experiences of women in medical academia. Bennett and

Nickerson (1992) surveyed female teaching and research faculty of the School of Physicians & Surgeons at Columbia University regarding perceived obstacles to advancement for women in academic medicine. Over 80 percent of the women surveyed reported conflicts between their personal and professional commitments and most of this group believed that their institution did not adequately address the needs of women with children. While half of those surveyed agreed that promotions were biased, one-third stated that sexist behavior was common and that sexual harassment occurred in their workplace. Findings from this study suggest that the structure or environment of medical academia may be non-supportive in several key areas and thereby detrimental to promotion and advancement of female faculty.

MINORITIES IN MEDICINE

Education of Minority Physicians

Historically, minority applicants to medical school have encountered formidable barriers. Up until the late 1960s medical education was segregated, formal and informal discriminatory policies and practices were commonplace, and financial support was unavailable (Shea and Fullilove 1985; Taylor et al. 1990; Petersdorf 1992; USDHHS 1993). Eighty-five percent of all underrepresented minority medical school students graduated from two traditionally black medical schools—Meharry and Howard. Before 1964, less than three percent of students entering medical schools were black—at that time the largest minority group in the U.S. (approximately ten percent of the population) (USDHHS 1993: 4).

During the late 1960s and early 1970s, a national commitment to equal opportunity, expressed through federal government affirmative action initiatives, brought about increased efforts of recruitment, admissions, and enrollment of minority (and female) students in the health professions. The Association of American Medical Colleges (AAMC) acknowledged that historic structural barriers and unequal educational preparation put blacks and other minorities at a competitive disadvantage with white students.

In 1970, the AAMC committed to the expansion of opportunities for minorities in medicine, established a goal to increase representation of underrepresented minorities in medical school to population parity, that is, 12 percent of the medical school population by 1975. The federal government as well as several foundations devoted substantial resources to this goal. Health professional schools joined forces with undergraduate colleges to provide programs and assistance to lift barriers limiting minority admission in health professional schools (Petersdorf et al. 1990; Epps, Cureton-Russell, and Kitzman 1993; USDHHS 1993).

In the period of 1964 to 1974, affirmative action policies dramatically increased the number of minority students entering American medical schools. By 1974, "underrepresented" minority enrollment (African Americans, American Indians, Mexican Americans, and mainland Puerto Ricans) reached a peak of 9.8 percent. Financial aid, tutorial, and enrichment programs assisted many of these students through medical school (Petersdorf et al. 1990).

From the mid-1970s to the early 1980s, the percentages of minority students entering medical school and programs supporting them steadily decreased. Several factors contributed to these declines. Federal government support for physician education halted in the 1980s as a result of the 1980 Graduate Medical Education National Advisory Council (GMENAC) projection of a physician surplus, even though GMENAC recommended that minority programs be continued. Early efforts to increase minority applicants to medical school were successful because they provided opportunities to an existing pool of qualified students who had previously been excluded by formal barriers. Challenges to affirmative action policies in the 1970s probably contributed to these declines as well (Shea and Fullilove 1985: 933).

Minority enrollment increased slightly again in the mid-1980s and again after 1990. By 1992, underrepresented minorities represented 12 percent of all first-year medical students. Although this is the largest proportion ever, it still does not meet population parity, which is about 16 percent (Petersdorf et al. 1990: 664). Graduation trends for underrepresented minorities remained steady in the 1980s, but in 1992 decreased slightly to eight percent of all graduates (USDHHS 1993: 5).

The low proportion of minority medical school graduates is of particular concern because demographic trends indicate that minority groups in the U.S. are becoming more heterogeneous and are growing at a faster rate than the majority population.[7] Cregler, Clark, and Jackson (1994) observe that the total applicant pool to U.S. medical schools declined after 1985, and for the first time, minority applicants decreased. The largest decrease was among African American males whose applicant pool was 39 percent lower in 1990 than it had been in 1974 (USDHHS 1993: 6). This trend is attributed to the decline in college enrollment and graduation of African Americans and other minorities. AAMC data indicate that, since 1990, despite improved academic credentials and MCAT scores, there appears to be a decrease in acceptance and matriculation rate of minority students relative to all other applicants. In 1975, 41 percent of minority compared to 39 percent of all other applicants were accepted compared to 51 percent and 59 percent, respectively, in 1990 (Petersdorf 1992: 76).

Both the U.S. Health Resources and Services Administration (HRSA) and the AAMC recognize that minority applicants face distinct barriers to medical education, namely, lack of financial support, inadequate educational preparation at all levels, and few role models (Petersdorf 1992; USDHHS 1993). Costs of medical education have increased steadily since 1983. In 1990, approximately ten percent of minority medical school graduates had no school debt compared to 20 percent of all other students. Approximately 80 percent of minority medical students had obtained scholarships compared to 49 percent of all other students. Minority students, however, were less likely than others to receive loans from family and friends (USDHHS 1993: 7). Financial indebtedness in medical school constrains career choices regarding specialty and type of practice. Advanced specialty training usually means more indebtedness. Financial indebtedness most likely propels young physicians who may not otherwise choose it into salaried practice arrangements (USDHHS 1993: 14).

College and graduate school entry rates are significantly lower for minority compared to white Americans. The AAMC has identified this as a major obstacle to enrolling minority applicants to medical school and has embarked on a series of programs to encourage medical schools to develop minority enrichment programs at the high school and college levels through a combination of public and private efforts (Petersdorf et al. 1990; USDHHS 1993: 6).

Several U.S. colleges and medical schools have incorporated programs that offer minority students science and math enrichment programs beginning in the elementary and secondary level in an effort to create an educational "pipeline" to minority enrollment in medical school (Petersdorf 1992). This relatively recent collaboration among educational institutions at various levels is viewed by many analysts as a model for education of minority students for careers in the health professions.

Close relationships with established professionals are cited as another important factor in the career advancement of minority students. In a longitudinal study of African Americans in professional schools, Blackwell (1987) found that the most powerful predictor of enrollment and graduation of blacks from professional schools is the presence of black faculty (1987: 359). Earlier research by Blackwell (1983) indicated that black students experienced problems in forming social networks on white campuses and were not likely to be selected as protégés by potential mentors. Other advocates (Peterson and Carlson 1992; Brewer, DuVal, and Davis 1979; Watts, Harris, and Pearson 1989; Thurmond and Mott 1990; Taylor et al. 1990; Cregler 1993; Cregler et al. 1994) cite the importance of minority role models and mentors for minority students in medical schools:

> Minority role models and mentors are essential to successful recruitment and maintenance of minorities in the biomedical sciences pipeline...mentor programs help students cope with the demands and stress of professional education...The mentor relationship is dynamic and important in fostering professional socialization (Cregler et al. 1994: 69).

Such observations suggest that, no less than in decades past, an informal system of professional guidance complements the formal system of medical education without which minority students will not be able to be fully integrated into the mainstream of the medical profession. Epps et al. (1993) undertook a systematic review of strategies and programs resulting from academic and community-based collaborations to increase minority enrollment in the health professions and found few published studies or evaluations that attempted to assess accomplishments. They identified three predominant strategies and programs—awareness, reinforcement/ enrichment, and prematriculation—which were applied across institutions, programs, and disciplines; consistently produced acceptable outcomes; and were endorsed by policy-making groups of the respective health profession. They concluded that such programs (which range from career awareness days to the establishment of health profession magnet schools) have been successful but have lacked guidance in standardizing outcomes, documenting, and publishing results (1993: 125).

Career Patterns of Minority Physicians

As noted earlier, minority and female medical graduates are significantly more likely than white males to practice primary care medicine. Babbott et al. (1989) point out that some minority graduates may end up practicing in primary care because of social or economic constraints rather than by choice. Their 1987 national study of U.S. medical school seniors found that minorities were matched to their first choice of residency program less than half as often as the national norm. Evidence suggests that there might, indeed, be a gap between desired and actual resident specialties. In 1990, 28 percent of minority medical school graduates indicated primary care medicine as their first choice, whereas in 1990, 43 percent of black and 46 percent of Hispanic residents actually practiced in primary care (USDHHS 1993: 12). Although these data represent two different cohorts of residents and, as such, are not causally related, they are indicative of a possible discrepancy between the specialty desired and actually practiced.

In a second study, Babbott, Weaver, and Baldwin (1994) analyzed AAMC data regarding specialty choices of 1983 graduating seniors and compared that to their first through third-year residency status to determine whether blacks and other underrepresented minority medical graduates enter primary care "by choice or by default." Although the vast majority of first-year residents (95 percent) did begin a program in their original specialty choice, minorities were significantly less likely to commence in a preferred specialty than were whites (3.5 percent of minorities vs. 1.7 percent of whites). The drop-out rate within the three years of residency training is particularly noteworthy. By the third year of training, only 77.5 percent of respondents were in the specialty they preferred as medical seniors and there were considerable differences by race/ethnicity. Despite the fact that white and Asian students tended to choose more competitive specialties within the "supporting services" (anesthesiology, pathology, radiology, rehabilitation medicine, public health/preventive medicine, emergency medicine) than all other groups, they were less likely than all other groups to have dropped their preferred specialty by the third year. Seventy-nine percent of Asian and 78 percent of white third-year residents were still in their senior year-preferred specialty compared to less than 66 percent of black third-year residents (Babbott et al. 1994).

Although this study does not probe the reasons for discrepancies in attrition in graduate training by race/ethnicity, the authors speculate that a variety of factors could be at work: medical school indebtedness influences some to drop out of specialty training and enter primary care by default as a means of earning a living; health problems; family and childrearing considerations; and perceived differences in clinical performance that make advancement within subspecialties more difficult (Babbott et al. 1994).

As noted in Chapter Two, physician practice setting characteristics differ by race/ethnicity. The 1987 AMA Young Physician Survey indicates that African American and Hispanic physicians are much more likely than whites to choose solo practice arrangements and much less likely than whites to choose group practice. Thirty percent of young black and 34 percent of young Hispanic physicians choose solo practice compared to about 25 percent of white physicians. Forty percent of young white physicians compared to under 20 percent of young black physicians and about 33 percent of young Hispanic physicians practice in groups. Over 50 percent of young black and about 33 percent of young Hispanic and white physicians practice in salaried arrangements (including HMOs, academic institutions, government hospital, private business, other physician, or other type of employer) (USDHHS 1993: 14). Some researchers suggest that anticipated peer or patient discrimination may discourage minority physicians from practicing in groups dominated by white physicians (Adams and Bazzolli 1986).

Minorities in Medical Academia

Minorities are far from being integrated into the mainstream of medical academia. According to the AAMC, underrepresented minority faculty represented 3.5 percent of the full-time medical school faculty in 1992 compared to 2.6 percent in 1982. Blacks comprised 65 percent of this minority faculty total. Yet, over one-third of these faculty members were located either at minority medical schools or at minority medical centers while holding faculty positions at majority medical schools (Wilson and Kaczmarek 1993: 97).

Data from the 1989 AAMC Faculty Roster indicate that among faculty with M.D. degrees, broad disparities exist between the proportions of minority faculty who hold professor or associate professor titles compared with other groups. Thirty-seven percent of underrepresented minority versus 53 percent of all others hold higher professional titles of professor or associate professor. Although these statistics were not controlled for age (the difference may reflect the fact that minority faculty are probably younger), it does appear that minority faculty are not promoted as quickly as others. On average, promotion of medical school faculty takes place within three to seven years. Forty-two percent of underrepresented minority faculty compared to 27 percent of all others took eight years or more to attain associate professor rank (Petersdorf et al. 1990). Possible reasons for the slower advancement of minority faculty could be the subtle discriminatory practices that Lorber (1984) has described.

Cregler et al. (1994) suggest that minority faculty are oftentimes placed into needed but less-valued positions within the academic hierarchy due to a combination of factors (such as administrative work, hospital and medical school committee assignments, and student counseling) which reduce time for research. In addition, they note that "the need to publish or perish may cause great conflict for minority faculty, who see the great service needs of their community, minority students, and house staff" (Cregler et al. 1994: 70). They cite multiple factors that probably account for the low proportionate numbers of minorities in academia: few minority medical school graduates, indebtedness of minority postgraduates, lack of awareness of opportunities in academic medical centers, lack of mentors and role models, and inadequate support systems to help minorities succeed in the academic arena (Cregler et al. 1994: 68).

Career Satisfaction

Research by Hadley et al. (1992) supports the suggestion that numerous factors adversely affect the careers of young minority and female physicians. They examined factors associated with career dissatisfaction among a sample of young physicians surveyed in 1987 by the AMA and found that, among the 19 percent of physicians who were "most likely to have second thoughts" about a career in medicine, there were significantly higher proportions of blacks, Hispanics, and white women compared to white men. These groups reported significantly higher educational indebtedness, more working hours per week, and lower incomes compared to white males.

The authors note that there are a few possible explanations for these findings. Medical school curricula and their social support systems may not be preparing students for the realities of medical practice, while school indebtedness may be creating serious impediments to successful medical careers, particularly for students from low income families. Finally, subtle discriminatory practices may limit the specialty choices and career opportunities of young women and minority physicians (1992: 188).

Hadley et al. stress that further research is needed to clarify the various factors at work, specifically, the processes through which women and minorities are encouraged or discouraged in practice:

> A better understanding is needed of how women and
> minority physicians in training may be steered toward or

away from particular specialty choices, or may be made
to feel uncomfortable participating in the full spectrum of
medical training opportunities (1992: 188-189).

They further speculate that the promotion of qualified minority and
female physicians within academic institutions may help break down
barriers that impede physicians in training (1992: 189).

INTERNATIONAL MEDICAL GRADUATES IN MEDICINE

Career Patterns of International Medical Graduates

Foreign-born status is closely linked with international medical
graduate status. International medical graduates (IMGs) have traditionally
functioned as a surplus labor pool in the United States to substitute in less
desirable positions unfilled by U.S. medical graduates (USMGs). In the
post-World War II era, the growth of public and private monies for
medical research opened up opportunities for international medical
graduates to pursue advanced study in the U.S. The presence of foreign
nationals in residency programs in the U.S. peaked in the early 1970s with
a high of 10,000, nearly 20 percent of the total number of graduate
medical trainees (Harrington et al. 1991).[8] During the period 1980 and
1992 the number of foreign-national IMGs entering practice increased
steadily. In 1992, foreign-national IMGs comprised almost 20 percent of
the active physicians in the U.S. (Mullan, Politzer, and Davis 1995).

The popular notion of IMGs as "cheap labor from poor nations" is
widespread within the medical literature (Torrey and Taylor 1973; Dublin
1974; Foreman 1990) which has tended to focus on concerns regarding
IMGs' lack of competence and the implications for the quality of health
care. Sociological studies (Fox and Richards 1977; Stevens, Goodman,
and Mick 1978; Mick and Lee 1997) have shown that IMGs function in
less desirable positions within the highly stratified system of the medical
profession, filling in vacancies in locations of high medical need.

Recent calls to restrict the entry and permanent residence of foreign-national IMGs in the U.S. include highly publicized reports by the Pew Health Professions Commission (1995) as well as the Institute of Medicine (1996). Both researchers and advocates within the profession point out that restriction of this particular group of physicians may have serious consequences (Stimmel 1996; Mick and Lee 1997). Stimmel argues that it is neither pragmatic nor morally acceptable to single out IMGs in an effort to decrease physician numbers in the U.S. Mick and Lee's analysis of 1996 data on all active postresident physicians in the U.S. found that IMGs tended to be overrepresented in counties of lower than average physician-to-population ratio or where there was high infant mortality, data which support the notion that IMGs practice in locations where USMGs will not.

Studies of IMGs' practice location patterns date back to the mid 1970s. Fox and Richards (1977) used correlational analyses in their study of physician distribution at the state level and found that practice locations of the more "dominant physicians" (that is, those who had been licensed, and therefore established, for a longer period of time) "are best predicted by affluence and urbanization" whereas practice locations of the least dominant physicians (IMGs and newly licensed MDs) are best predicted by job availability" (1977: 366).[9] In other words, more dominant physicians tended to locate in economically rewarding areas, whereas less dominant physicians tended to locate around available less rewarding job openings. This concept of dominance is consistent with the notion of marginalization of certain groups of physicians into less desirable positions within the profession.

In a 1974 survey of interns and residents in the AMA-approved training programs in American hospitals, Stevens et al. (1978) found that IMGs filled residual roles in the American medical system, taking vacant positions in hospitals, locations, and specialties. They note that informal processes of education in the American medical system inhibit the complete socialization of IMGs into the mainstream of American medicine. IMGs as a group enter less prestigious positions than USMGs and this point of entry into the profession determines much of their later experience. IMGs may have little contact with USMGs during their training and have cultural and often language barriers that may hamper their socialization as American physicians. In general, they are given less professional responsibility with patients than are U.S. trained physicians. Stevens et al. note that this results in less clinical autonomy and overall a "less complete apprentice-ship" than USMGs receive (1978: 180-181).

Stevens et al. also observe that within the IMG pool there is further stratification: women are less upwardly mobile than men; Asians are less mobile than those who are culturally most like Americans, namely U.S. national IMGs and other English speakers (1978: 157). They conclude that these patterns most likely reflect "cultural competence" as opposed to "technical competence," that is, the most successful IMGs are those who possessed auxiliary statuses that eased their transition and enabled them to assimilate into the American medical profession. They note that:

> cultural competence...is a critical gateway to other forms of learning. The resident who is not perceived as a 'full' physician has fewer opportunities for informal discussions and consultations and is given less clinical responsibility...Thus the physician who is regarded as less 'competent' may, in the end, be less competent by having a lesser education (1978: 205).

By not receiving proper institutional support—that is, organizational and cultural orientation, ample collegial interaction, and opportunities to exercise clinical judgement—IMGs are set up to fail. Thus the IMG becomes a classic example of the self-fulfilling prophecy (Merton 1957: 421-436) and is thereby marginalized into a less desirable position within the profession.

Mick's (1987) analysis of Stevens et al.'s data indicates that IMGs were significantly more likely than USMGs to enter lower-prestige hospitals and to enter low-prestige medical practices. Mick also found an additive effect: namely, residents from low-prestige hospitals were significantly more likely to enter low-prestige practices. He observes that the "Matthew effect" and the "Salieri phenomenon" are two forces that may explain the status distinctions perpetuated between IMGs and

USMGs. Mick notes that these two processes also operate at an organizational level to maintain status distinctions between training hospitals and types of medical practice. He concludes:

> FMGs lack an American 'old boy' network, sponsorship leading to visibility and testimonials of competence, and an open jury system which counters the accumulation of advantage via the Matthew effect. Whatever sponsorship occurs tends to resemble Salieri's backhanded promotion of Mozart...performance goes unnoticed or is undervalued, resulting in a smaller share of rewards, and so diminished achieved status is linked with devalued ascribed status (1987: 83).

By Stonequist's definition, foreign-born international medical graduates appear to be a prototype of the marginal person. As professionals, they fit Hughes' categorization of the marginal professional with a status dilemma. Caught between the medical system in which they were educated and the one in which they work, the IMG does not belong completely to either. Stevens et al. argue that placement of international medical school graduates into needed but marginal positions in the U.S. medical profession takes place through an elaborate mechanism of social control. They note:

> The stereotype of the foreign-trained physician...who practices substandard medicine fits very well with the need to place FMGs in permanent positions less desired by American trained physicians. The stereotypes contribute to an ideology that makes it easy to continue...to place (FMGs) in less desired situations in the...medical manpower market or to discontinue their use entirely on grounds of 'quality' when the supply of American graduates changes (1978: 271).

Licensure is viewed as an indicator of physician competence in the United States. In addition to the manifest function of licensing (to protect citizens from poor quality of care) sociological theory suggests that latent functions also exist. Social functions of licensing include: control of numbers of practitioners; allocation of personnel to practice settings, status levels, and specialties; expression of social values (for example, values regarding the integration or segregation of newcomers into the larger society); and finally the maintenance of professional elitism (Shuval 1985).

Goldblatt et al. (1975) observe that licensure may not be an accurate indicator of IMG physician competence and that, rather, it serves latent functions. Using a national sample of interns and residents trained in 1963, they compared 1971 licensure rates for USMGs and IMGs and found wide disparities: over 30 percent of IMGs were unlicensed compared to seven percent of USMGs. In examining associated factors, they found that visa or citizenship status and state of examination—conditions unrelated to competence—were strong predictors of licensure, whereas quality of medical education was not an accurate predictor of licensure. They observe that "exchange-visitor" visa status is an almost certain barrier to obtaining a U.S. medical license and that different states vary widely in their licensing rates of IMGs. Goldblatt et al. suggest that this phenomenon is most likely related to personnel needs of the individual states:

> The strategy of attracting large numbers of FMGs, licensing relatively few of them, and requiring the unlicensed FMGs to work in certain institutions could allow certain states to ease the critical shortage of physicians needed in hospitals. One statistical artifact that would result from such a strategy would be a high proportion of unlicensed FMGs (1975: 140).

Goldblatt et al.'s study suggests that licensing rates are not good measures of physician competence and consequently, quality of medical care. Hospital positions oftentimes do not require licenses, and IMGs working in hospitals may therefore not seek them (Goldblatt et al. 1975:

140). It appears that international medical graduates function to relieve physician shortages in medically underserved areas, and barriers to licensure limit their movement away from institutions in these areas.

The label "incompetent," so often attached to IMGs, lends justification to continued distinctions between U.S. and foreign-trained physicians. In a review of studies of IMG performance, Tan (1977) contends that serious flaws such as nonblind studies, possible bias in peer reviews, small sample sizes, and poor scaling of measures lend serious doubt to studies' negative findings regarding IMG competencies. According to Tan:

> Elimination of restrictive, discriminatory procedures and regulations aimed at the foreign graduate, vastly improved orientation techniques, and the elimination of training programs that exploit the foreign medical graduate solely as cheap labor can improve assimilation of foreign physicians into the American health care system (1977: 828).

Barriers to licensure in the 1990s still vary by states, whose boards of medical examiners may place additional requirements on IMGs beyond those required of USMGs (Myers 1995). Anecdotal information corroborates the suggestion that there is still widespread formal as well as informal discrimination. One physician described what appears to be a common experience among IMGs:

> After you get into practice, you keep hearing stories of people who either get turned down for promotions, or don't get faculty appointments, or have problems in their medical societies because they're from foreign schools (Myers 1995: 31).

There are indications that IMGs are acutely sensitive to issues related to their professional competencies. In a 1973 national study of U.S. physicians, Colombotos, Charles, and Kirchner (1977) found that IMGs exhibited more liberal attitudes than USMGs toward a variety of government in health issues except one—they were significantly less likely than USMGs (34 percent vs. 52 percent) to favor peer reviews of physicians' work. Peer review involves formal assessments by physicians in hospitals and other work settings and inclusion of such assessments in state or federal regulations. They conclude that IMGs may respond unfavorably to reviews because they perceive them as more professionally threatening than do their USCG counterparts (1977: 606).

Despite recent efforts to restrict their arrival and permanent residence, it appears that IMGs have begun the process of integration within the American medical profession. Their growing influence is evidenced by the formation of a section within the AMA focused on IMGs' specific issues as well as the formation of professional associations of IMGs in individual states (Mick and Lee 1997).

CONCLUSION

Empirical studies indicate that women, minority, and foreign-born and foreign-educated physicians are more likely than other physicians to care for larger numbers of low-income patients. Previous studies of physician participation in Medicaid emphasize the economic motivations that dominate physicians' decisions to accept Medicaid patients. This chapter has argued that structural constraints on the professional choices of female, minority, and foreign-born, foreign-educated physicians are also determinants of Medicaid participation. Chapter Four outlines the data, methods, and measurements used for the analysis of this study.

NOTES

1. Many studies of physician supply in the U.S. distinguish between "underrepresented minorities" those minority physicians who are underrepresented within the medical profession proportionate to their numbers in the overall population (In 1990, Latinos were 4.9 percent of the physician population and 9 percent of the U.S. population; African Americans are 3.6 percent of all physicians and 11.7 percent of the U.S. population; American Indians are 0.1 percent of the physician population and 1 percent of the U.S. population) and those minority physicians who are overrepresented (In 1990, Asians and Asian Americans were 11.8 percent of the physician population and 2.8 percent of the U.S. population) (USDHHS 1993: i). The AAMC further distinguishes among Hispanics, considering only Mexican Americans and mainland Puerto Ricans as "underrepresented" in medicine (Babbott et al. 1989).

2. Results from this study also indicated that white female and minority male residents' specialty patterns were beginning to approximate those of white men, whereas minority women were significantly more likely than the other three groupings to plan practices in traditionally female specialties of pediatrics and obstetrics/gynecology (Adams and Bazzoli 1986: 18). This pattern may be an indication that white women and minority males are slowly being integrated into many levels of mainstream medicine, whereas minority women are still marginalized within less prestigious specialties and positions. It is unclear, however, whether this is a long-term trend.

3. Historians and sociologists of science have fostered the notion of the "marginal scientist as innovator" in the public imagination. Scientific lore is filled with accounts of the obscure practitioner who unexpectedly contributes to basic medical research, and the lone scientist in a backwater institution estranged from the institutional centers of scientific research (Merton 1973: 518-519).

Merton's notion of membership encompassed the marginal man as a type of nonmember, the "ineligible aspirant" (1957: 290). Cole (1979) characterized women scientists as historically "marginal" to the larger scientific community. Close relatives to the marginal man are Simmel's and Camus' depictions of the "stranger."

4. In their examination of "the marginal scientist" as the prototypical innovator in science, Gieryn and Hirsh concluded that the manner in which marginality had been operationalized was lacking. They scrutinized the careers of innovators in the field of X-ray astronomy and found little support for the notion that scientific innovation comes more often from the margin rather than the center. However defined, marginal scientists were no more likely to provide innovation in research than nonmarginal scientists. They observe that "the ideas of 'marginality' and 'innovation' are caught up in many conceptual cobwebs" (102) and conclude that "the concept of marginality is, in its present use, so ambiguous as to be almost worthless as a conceptual tool for systematic inquiry into the sources of scientific innovation" (Gieryn and Hirsh 1983: 87).

5. This term originates from words attributed to Christ in the Gospel according to Matthew: "For whosoever hath, to him shall be given, and he shall have more abundance: but whosoever hath not, from him shall be taken away even that he hath" (Matthew Chapter 25 Verse 29).

6. In 1991, less than 10 percent of female faculty (1,463) held the rank of full professor compared to 32 percent of male faculty (16,841); 20 percent of women and 25 percent of men held associate professor titles; 50 percent of women compared to 35 percent of men held assistant professor titles (Bickel and Kopriva 1993).

7. The proportion of minority school-age children in the U.S. population, for example, is expected to grow from 20 percent in 1985 to 33 percent by the year 2000 (Petersdorf et al. 1990: 665).

8. The Council on Graduate Medical Education (COGME) established by the U.S. Congress advised the executive branch on several aspects of policy, one of the results being a more restrictive policy on the participation of IMGs in graduate medical education (Council on Graduate Medical Education. *First Report of the Council. Vol 1.* Washington, D.C.: U.S. Department of Health and Human Services, 1988).

9. The authors employ the concept of "physician dominance" developed by Freidson (1970). Freidson discussed physician dominance as the power of physicians over other types of health workers and patients, rooted in the profession's monopolization of technological and scientific knowledge. Fox and Richards extend this notion of dominance to include "inter-physician" types.

IV

Methods and Measurements

SAMPLING AND DATA COLLECTION

This study is a secondary analysis of physician data from Colombotos and colleagues' 1990 nationwide survey of physicians and nurses (Colombotos et al. 1995). The sampling design, questionnaire design and data collection were carried out in collaboration with the National Opinion Research Center (NORC) at the University of Chicago.

Data for the 1990 study were collected specifically to assess physicians' and nurses' AIDS-related knowledge, attitudes, and practices; however, a question regarding physicians' Medicaid participation was used for the present analysis. Data for 958 physicians were collected by telephone interview and mail questionnaire between July 1990 and January 1991.

Respondents were selected from a two-stage national probability sample of all physicians in twenty-five states stratified by geographic region and cumulative AIDS rate with oversampling of physicians in San Francisco and New York City. The 25 states were sampled with a probability proportionate to the combined number of physicians and nurses in each state. The sample was then weighted to take into account the higher selection probabilities of New York City and San Francisco respondents. In calculating sample weights, New York City and San Francisco respondents were weighted downward. The sample weights were multiplied by a constant so that the weighted number of cases equalled the weighted eligible total of 958 physicians. Appendix I contains an abstracted technical description of the sampling design by NORC.

The physician sample was drawn from the American Medical Association's Physician Masterfile, which includes all licensed physicians in the United States, and was restricted to physicians whose primary specialty was listed as family practice, general practice, internal medicine and its subspecialties, pediatrics, general surgery, other surgical specialty, or obstetrics-gynecology. The sample was limited to the 958 physicians who indicated that they had spent a minimum of 10 hours per week in direct patient care in that specialty during the previous 12 months.

RESPONSE RATES

After three months of data collection efforts, the response rate of physicians in the survey was 47 percent (704 completed interviews from an eligible sample of 1,505—referred to as "Phase I" of the survey). A strategy[1] was developed to upgrade the response rate by choosing a random sample of one-half of the 801 nonrespondents and following them up with an alternative approach, namely, a mailed self-administered questionnaire and a $25.00 check. Questionnaires or telephone interviews were completed with 254 of the 401 physicians within the next 13 weeks, referred to as "Phase II" of the survey (Table 4.1). The 254 cases were double-weighted and added to the other completed 704 cases for a weighted total of 1,212 completed cases out of 1,505—a weighted response rate of 80 percent.[2]

Table 4.1   Respondents by Phase and Mode[1]

Mode	Phase I		Phase II		Total	
	N	%	N	%	N	%
Telephone	679	96	22	9	701	73
Mail	25	4	232	91	257	27
Total	704	100	254	100	958	100

[1]Figures in this table are not weighted

WEIGHTING OF SAMPLE

Unless otherwise noted, all figures in this study are appropriately weighted as previously described. The adjusted figures reflect estimates of various statistics for probability samples of physicians practicing in the U.S. during the period 1989 to 1990.

TYPES AND SOURCES OF DATA GATHERED

Data from the 1990 national survey provided information on physician background characteristics (gender, racial or ethnic minority status, and foreign or U.S. birthplace), professional characteristics (foreign or U.S. medical school, medical specialty and board certification status) and practice characteristics (practice setting and practice location by zipcode). It also provided measures of physicians' political and professional ideology, and physicians' estimates of the percentage of their patient population on Medicaid.

Data from the 1990 U.S. Census was used to characterize physician practice location at the zipcode level by percentage minority population and poverty rate. These measures provide a means by which to assess the relationship of salient local service area characteristics to physician participation in Medicaid.

MEASURES

The major dependent variable in this research is "Medicaid patient population." The measure is based on individual physicians' responses to the question: "About what percentage of your patients are covered by Medicaid?" Responses ranged from zero to 100 percent. The same or similar question ("About what percentage of your patients have Medicaid?") was used in other national surveys of physicians (Mitchell and Cromwell 1980; Perloff et al. 1987).

The answer to this question was based on physicians' self-reports, and as such, under- or over-reporting is a potential source of error. In an attempt to assess self-reporting bias, Kletke et al. (1985) compared office-based pediatricians' self-reports regarding Medicaid participation with aggregated patient records and found that the pediatricians did, in fact, overestimate the extent of their Medicaid participation compared to patient records. The two measures of Medicaid participation, however, were highly correlated (Pearson's r = +.77; p < .001). The authors concluded that either measure can be used to accurately identify the determinants of physician Medicaid participation. It is conceivable that there could be error in the sampling of patient records; however, to the extent that the sample of patient records is representative, it can be used to gauge the accuracy of the doctors' estimates of Medicaid participation.

Review of Conceptual Definitions

The independent variables used in this study include the following measures:

Social marginality, discussed in Chapters Two and Three, is a condition associated with long-standing social barriers. Women, racial and ethnic minorities, and foreigners are social groups that historically have been discriminated against and "marginal" to the U.S. medical profession. Although some analysts make distinctions between "underrepresented" and "overrepresented" minorities in the medical profession, I chose to group them both into a single category "minority" and compare them to white, non-Hispanics (see Appendix II). My rationale for this grouping is that any racial or ethnic minority group is, by definition, a socially marginal status within the medical profession.

Social marginality includes physician racial/ethnic minority status (white non-Hispanic versus all other), birthplace (U.S. versus foreign), and gender (male versus female). In regression analyses, social marginality variables are scored as dummy variables with values of 0 or 1.

Professional marginality may be conceptualized as less desirable and prestigious statuses in the U.S. medical profession. Marginal professional statuses are expected to result from, and be closely linked to, marginal social statuses. The professional statuses considered are also those that are associated with Medicaid participation.

Marginal professional statuses include: practice setting (institutional vs. solo and group practice), place of medical school (U.S. vs. foreign), medical specialty (pediatrics vs. all others), board certification status (board-certified vs. no board certification) [see Appendix II]. In regression analyses, these are scored as dummy variables with values of 0 or 1.

Two other professional marginality variables included in this analysis are the 1990 U.S. Census poverty rate and the percent minority population for physicians' practice locations' zipcode areas. I have labelled them "practice characteristics." Appendix III contains the formulas used to calculate percentages for these variables from population counts. Values for these two variables range from zero to 100 percent.

Ideology consists of two variables:

1) *political ideology*—based on responses to the question: "In your political thinking, do you consider yourself...very liberal, liberal, middle-of-the-road, conservative, or very conservative?" scored on a five-point Likert scale, and

2) *professional ideology*—a scale consisting of nine questions in which physicians were asked if specific groups of physicians and nurses were professionally obligated and should be legally required to treat HIV patients. (Cronbach's standardized item alpha = .93 for the nine-item scale) Responses to these questions—agree strongly, agree somewhat, disagree somewhat, disagree strongly—were scored on a four-point Likert scale.[3]

In lieu of a more precise measure, the "obligation to treat HIV patients" is considered an indicator of a sense of obligation to treat stigmatized patients in general, including Medicaid patients. Fredericks, Munday and Kosa (1974) provided evidence from a national sample of physicians to suggest that one aspect of physicians' professional ideology is a "socially conscious orientation," or a service dimension. I posit that the "obligation to treat" scale measures this socially conscious orientation.

Exploratory factor analysis extracted one substantively meaningful factor on nine items using the maximum likelihood method (see Table 4.2). Scale items had been standardized in the Colombotos et al. study (see Appendix IV) with values ranging from -1.69 to +1.11.

Table 4.2   Factor Analysis of Obligation to Treat Scale[1,2]

Variable	Factor 1
Legally required to provide care:	
T1. physicians in their office practice	0.540
T2. attending physicians in hospital	0.554
T3. surgeons	0.573
T4. registered nurses in hospital	0.543
Professionally unethical to refuse care:	
T5. for you, yourself	0.827
T6. physicians in their office practice	0.877
T7. attending physicians in hospital	0.924
T8. surgeons	0.876
T9. registered nurses in hospital	0.890

[1] See also Appendix II (Study Measures—Scale Items and Reliabilities) and Appendix IV (Scale Construction)

[2] Figures are unweighted.

ANALYSIS OF THE EFFECTS OF PHASE AND MODE OF INTERVIEW

Since physicians were interviewed by both telephone and mail in two phases, the effects of mode of data collection and "early" versus "late" respondents should be considered. Mode and phase of interview are highly correlated (Pearson's $r = .879$; $p < .001$); most of the telephone interviews took place in the early phase of the study.

Weighted correlations of major study variables with phase and mode indicate that early telephone respondents reported higher percentages of Medicaid patients in their practices than later mail respondents. Initially, it might appear as though telephone respondents overestimated their participation in Medicaid compared to mail respondents. However, several other major independent variables were also significantly correlated with phase and mode of interview. Females, pediatricians, and those practicing in institutional settings, high minority population and high poverty practice locations, and those expressing greater obligation to treat were significantly more likely to be among the early telephone respondents.

It is quite likely that the overrepresentation of physicians with higher Medicaid caseloads among the early telephone respondents is due, not to reporting bias, but rather to the fact that the early telephone respondents were those who do in fact tend to treat greater numbers of Medicaid patients. Early respondents were very likely physicians who were more favorably inclined towards the subject matter (Health Care Workers and AIDS) of the survey.

Because of the significant bivariate relationships found between phase and mode with the major study variables, I controlled for their effects in the regression analyses reported in Chapter Six. Phase and mode did not, however, significantly change the relationship of any of the independent variables to the dependent variable.

ANALYSIS OF RESPONSE RATES AND MISSING DATA

An analysis of nonrespondents in the national survey by Colombotos et al. (1995) indicated that there were no significant differences between respondents and nonrespondents on characteristics available in the AMA file, namely: gender, age, specialty, U.S. or international medical school graduate status, board certification, and "self-employed" status.

Approximately eight percent of physicians did not respond to the question "About what percentage of your patients are covered by Medicaid?" An analysis of responders and nonresponders to this question indicates that there were no significant differences between them with respect to the major demographic variables of race/ethnicity, birthplace, gender, medical specialty and U.S. or international medical (IMG) graduate status. Nonresponders, however, were significantly more likely than responders to practice in institutional settings and to not be board-certified (Table 4.3).

Table 4.3 Comparison of Responders and Nonresponders to the
Dependent Variable[1] with Respect to Other Factors[2]

	Responders (N=880) %	Nonresponders (N=79) %	Significance level
Female Gender	14	15	ns
Minority Race	19	17	ns
Foreign Born	20	24	ns
IMG	21	29	ns
Not Board Certified	25	36	$p < .05$
Institutional Practice Setting	17	32	$p < .001$

[1] "About what percentage of your patients are covered by Medicaid?"
[2] All figures are weighted.

NOTES

1. This strategy is described in: Deming, 1960: 68, 106-109; Madow, Nisselson, and Olkin, 1983: 72-73; and Groves, 1989:159-183.

2. The rationale for this strategy is described in the references in footnote 1.

3. In preliminary analyses for this study, I found that the legal and ethical obligation to treat scales in the Colombotos et al. study (1990) were positively correlated (Pearson's $r = .47$, $p < .001$). Each scale also showed significant positive correlations with the dependent variable "approximately what percentage of your patients are covered by Medicaid?" (legal obligation, Pearson's $r = .21$, $p < .001$; ethical obligation, Pearson's $r = .16$, $p < .001$).

Preliminary analyses that entered both scales separately into the same regression equation showed that the effect of each scale on the dependent variable was diminished by the effect of the other. Rather than drop one of the scales for my analysis, I chose to combine them into one measure. My rationale for this decision was that more, rather than fewer, items make for a more conceptually coherent and reliable scale. Factor analyses (Table 4.2) indicate that there is one underlying factor for all nine scale items. Cronbach's Alpha for the nine-item scale is .93.

V

A Social, Professional, and Ideological Profile of Physicians

INTRODUCTION

This chapter examines the social and professional characteristics as well as the ideology of physicians surveyed in 1990. It describes the relationships among marginal social statuses (female, minority, and foreign-born), professional statuses (country of medical school education, specialty, board certification, practice setting) and characteristics (percent minority population and poverty practice location), and physician ideology (political and professional).

The relationships among physicians' social and professional statuses and their political and professional ideologies were discussed in Chapter Two. It observed that the social origins and professional characteristics of physicians are continuing sources of socialization that affect their political and professional ideologies. Chapter Three reviewed the literature on the relationships between social and professional characteristics of physicians. It noted that some combinations of characteristics or "status-sets" (e.g. white, male neurosurgeon) are more frequent than others (black, female neurosurgeon). Specific social statuses, thus, appear to influence career statuses.

The social and professional characteristics of physicians are interesting from both theoretical and policy standpoints. Theoretically, it is interesting to understand the mechanisms by which physicians' status-sets and status-

sequences are patterned and predictable. Policywise, an understanding of
the barriers to advancement within the profession for women and minority
physicians is key to effective elimination of those obstacles.

SOCIAL STATUSES, PROFESSIONAL STATUSES AND IDEOLOGY

This section first examines physicians' social and professional statuses
in relation to each other; secondly, it describes the relationships among
multiple marginal social statuses and professional characteristics; and
finally, it examines the interrelationships among clusters of professional
characteristics and political and professional ideology.

Relationships Among Social and Professional Statuses

The following physicians in this survey were classified as "marginal":
all females, all minorities, and all physicians who were foreign-born. Less
than one-third of the physicians in this study had one or more of these
marginal characteristics. The remaining physicians with no marginal
characteristics (those who were males and white, non-Hispanic and U.S.
born) were classified as "dominant" physicians (Table 5.1).

Table 5.1   Physician Social Status[1]

STATUS	(N=958) %
Physicians with one or more marginal statuses	32
Physicians with no marginal statuses	64
Not Classified (missing data)	4

[1] All figures are weighted.

Fourteen percent of all physicians surveyed were female, 18 percent were racial or ethnic minorities, and 20 percent were foreign-born. Seven percent of the total group identified themselves as Hispanic or black— underrepresented minorities. Subgroups within the minority category (Hispanic, black non-Hispanic, Filipino, Asian/Pacific Islander, or other minority) were so small that further analyses would not be generalizable to the universe of physicians in the United States (Table 5.2).

Table 5.2 Physician Racial/Ethnic Background[1]

PHYSICIAN RACE/ETHNICITY	(N=958) %
White, Non-Hispanic	78
Black, Non-Hispanic	3
Hispanic	4
Filipino	3
Asian / Pacific Islander	6
Other	2
Missing Data	4

[1] All figures are weighted.

Upon closer examination, we see that female, minority, foreign-born and international medical graduate status are overlapping categories within this physician population. For example, 32 percent of all female physicians were foreign-born compared to only 18 percent of male physicians (p < .001). The vast majority of foreign-born physicians were also international medical graduates (IMGs). Eighty-three percent of foreign-born physicians compared to only five percent of U.S. born physicians were IMGs (p < .001).

Minority physicians were significantly more likely than white, non-Hispanic physicians to be female, foreign-born and to have graduated from a medical school outside of the U.S. (Table 5.3). Sixty-four percent of all

Table 5.3   Female, Foreign-born, and International Medical Graduate
             Physicians by Racial/Ethnic Status[1]

SOCIAL STATUS	White Non-Hispanic (N=749) %	Minority (N=173) %
Female	12	25***
Foreign-born	6	64***
International Medical Graduate	11	67***

[1] All figures are weighted.
*** p≤ .001

minority physicians in this study were foreign-born IMGs. Conversely,
only 23 percent of all minority physicians were U.S. born U.S. medical
school graduates (USMGs).

   Marginal (female, minority or foreign-born) and dominant (male, white
non-Hispanic, and U.S. born) physicians are compared with respect to
their professional characteristics in Table 5.4. Female, minority and
foreign-born physicians were overrepresented in pediatrics and
underrepresented in the surgical specialties. Specialty differences between
female and dominant physicians are especially striking. One out of four
women physicians surveyed were pediatricians compared to less than one
out of ten dominant physicians; fewer than one in ten female physicians
were surgeons compared to almost one in three dominant physicians.

   Dominant physicians were significantly more likely than marginal
physicians to be board-certified in one or more medical specialties. About
eight out of ten dominant physicians reported that they were board-
certified compared to about seven out of ten female and about six out of
ten minority and foreign-born physicians. (It should be noted, however,
that pediatricians were significantly more likely to be board-certified than

Table 5.4   Physician Professional Statuses and Characteristics by Social Status[1,2]

STATUS	(1) % of all Dominant MDs (N=611)	(2) % of all Female MDs (N=132)	(3) % of all Minority MDs (N=173)	(4) % of all Foreign-born MDs (N=191)
Specialty:				
Pediatrics	9	25***	15*	14*
FPGP	21	24	22	19
IM	30	33	36	34
ObGyn	7	11	7	7
Surgery	32	7***	20***	26+
Board-certified	81	69***	59***	60***
Setting:				
Institution	13	40***	26***	20*
Partner /Group	49	30***	23***	24***
Solo	37	30+	51***	56***

[1] All figures are weighted.

[2] Due to rounding, figures do not add up to 100%.

The following symbols indicate the level of statistical significance of differences between Groups 2,3,4 versus 1:

***   indicates a difference between Group 2,3, or 4 vs. Group 1 at $p \leq .001$

*   indicates a difference between Group 2,3, or 4 vs. Group 1 at $p \leq .01$

+   indicates a difference between Group 2,3, or 4 vs. Group 1 at $p \leq .10$

other specialists: 86 percent of pediatricians were board-certified in one or more specialty compared to 73 percent of all other specialists [p < .001].) Country of medical school was also closely linked to board-certification status. Only 56 percent of IMGs were board-certified in one or more medical specialties compared with 80 percent of USMGs (p < .001).

Marginal physicians, especially women, were disproportionately represented in institutional practice settings compared to dominant physicians. Forty percent of female, 26 percent of minority, and 20 percent of foreign-born physicians practiced in hospitals or other institutional settings compared to approximately 13 percent of dominant physicians. Dominant physicians were most heavily concentrated in partnership and group practices. Almost one-half of all dominant physicians practiced in partnership or group practices compared to one out of three females, and less than one out of four minority and foreign-born physicians.

All three types of marginal physicians were significantly more likely than dominant physicians to practice medicine in locations with high percentages of minority populations (Table 5.5). In addition, minority and foreign-born physicians were significantly more likely than dominant physicians to practice medicine in locations with high poverty populations.

All three groups of marginal physicians displayed a tendency toward greater political liberalism compared to dominant physicians on a five-point scale ranging from very conservative to very liberal (Table 5.5). Only female physicians, however, were significantly more likely than all other groups of physicians to label themselves as politically liberal (p < .001). Thirty-eight percent of all female, 19 percent of all minority, 21 percent of all foreign-born and 19 percent of non-Hispanic white, male U.S. born physicians identified as liberal in their politics. All three marginal groups of physicians also expressed a significantly greater obligation to treat stigmatized patients compared to dominant physicians.

Table 5.5   Physician Practice Location Characteristics and Political and
Professional Ideology by Social Status[1]

STATUS	(1) All Dominant MDs (N=611)	(2) All Female MDs (N=132)	(3) All Minority MDs (N=173)	(4) All Foreign-born MDs (N=191)
Mean % Minority Population of Practice Location	21.6	31.0***	39.4***	33.3***
Mean Poverty Rate of Practice Location	13.5	15.1	17.2***	15.5*
Mean Score Political Liberalism	2.68	3.16***	2.94***	2.91**
Mean Score Obligation to Treat	-0.49	-0.11***	-0.17***	-0.12***

[1] All figures are weighted..

The following symbols indicate the level of statistical significance of differences between Groups 2,3,4 versus 1:

*** indicates a difference between Group 2,3, or 4 vs. Group 1
at $p \leq .001$

* * indicates a difference between Group 2,3, or 4 vs. Group 1
at $p \leq .01$

* indicates a difference between Group 2,3, or 4 vs. Group 1
at $p \leq .05$

Effects of Multiple Marginal Social Statuses

In order to examine the effects of multiple marginal social statuses on professional statuses, physicians in the sample were grouped by the number of marginal social statuses they possessed (Table 5.6). Seventeen percent of physicians possessed one marginal status, 12 percent possessed two marginal statuses, and three percent possessed three marginal statuses.

As noted earlier, the data indicate that marginal social statuses are overlapping. In other words, some status-sets (foreign-born, minority female IMG) within the medical profession are more common than others (foreign-born, white male IMG). This fact raises the question of whether physicians possessing more marginal social statuses also possess more marginal professional statuses compared to physicians with fewer marginal social statuses; that is, does the fact that a physician possesses more marginal social statuses increase the likelihood that she or he will also possess more marginal professional statuses?

Table 5.6   Physicians by Number of Marginal Statuses[1]

NUMBER OF MARGINAL STATUSES	(N=958) %
No Marginal Social Statuses (Dominant MDs)	64
One Marginal Social Status	17
Two Marginal Social Statuses	12
Three Marginal Social Statuses	3
Not Classified (missing data)	4

[1] All figures are weighted.

Preliminary analyses for this study indicated that physicians who possessed three marginal statuses (female, minority, IMGs) were distinctive in that they occupied more professionally marginal statuses and characteristics than the other three groups of physicians. The number of physicians in this group (N=33), however, was too small to detect statistically meaningful differences compared to physicians with no, one or two marginal statuses. Therefore, for analytic purposes they were grouped together with physicians with two marginal statuses (Table 5.7).

The figures in Table 5.7 indicate that physicians with two or three marginal statuses were significantly less likely than physicians with no marginal statuses and those with one marginal status to be U.S. medical school graduates and to be board-certified in one or more medical specialties. They were significantly more likely than physicians with no marginal statuses (but equally likely as those with one marginal status) to practice in pediatrics and significantly less likely to practice in a surgical specialty. Also, physicians with two or three marginal social statuses were significantly more likely to be practicing in institutional settings compared to those with no marginal statuses but significantly less likely than those with one marginal status to be in institutional settings.

The figures in Table 5.8 indicate that physicians with two or three marginal social statuses were significantly more likely to be practicing in high minority population and high poverty locations compared to those with no or one marginal status. On average, physicians with two or three marginal statuses practiced in locations with almost 38 percent minority population and roughly 17 percent poverty rate, compared with almost 31 percent minority population and 14 percent poverty rate for those physicians with one marginal status, and an approximately 22 percent minority population and almost 14 percent poverty rate for physicians with no marginal statuses.

Physicians with two or three marginal statuses were significantly more likely than physicians with no marginal statuses (but equally as likely as those with one marginal status) to identify themselves as politically liberal. They were significantly more likely than physicians with no marginal statuses and those with one marginal status to express a greater obligation to treat stigmatized patients.

Table 5.7   Physician Medical School, Board Certification, Specialty and
            Practice Setting by Number of Marginal Social Statuses[1]

STATUS	(1) No Marginal Statuses (N=611) %	(2) One Marginal Status (N=164) %	(3) Two or Three Marginal Statuses (N=145) %
US Medical Graduate:	95	71***	20***
Board- certified	81	64***	61
Specialty:			
Pediatrics	9	18**	15
Surgery	32	23**	18*
Institutional Practice Setting:	13	33**	23**

[1] All figures are weighted.
*** p ≤ .001 (Group 2 vs. Group 1) (Group 3 vs. Group 2)
 ** p ≤ .01 (Group 2 vs. Group 1)
  * p ≤ .05 (Group 3 vs. Group 2)

Table 5.8   Physician Practice Location Characteristics and Ideology
by Number of Marginal Social Statuses[1]

STATUS	(1) No Marginal Statuses (N=611)	(2) One Marginal Status (N=164)	(3) Two or Three Marginal Statuses (N=145)
Mean % Minority Population of Practice Location	21.6	30.6***	37.5***
Mean Poverty Rate of Practice Location	13.5	14.2*	17.2***
Mean Score Political Liberalism	2.68	3.27***	2.86***
Mean Score Obligation to Treat	-0.49	-0.23***	-0.1*

[1] All figures are weighted.

*** $p \leq .001$ (Group 2 vs. Group 1) (Group 3 vs. Group 2)

  * $p \leq .05$ (Group 3 vs. Group 2)

Relationships Among Professional Characteristics and Physician Ideology

Several other groups of variables in this study are empirically linked. The correlation matrix (Table 5.9) indicates that certain marginal professional characteristics are highly correlated with each other: high minority population and high poverty practice locations are correlated categories ($r = .671$, $p < .001$); and institutionally-based practice setting is closely linked to both high minority population ($r = .281$, $p < .001$) and high poverty practice locations ($r = .262$, $p < .001$). Physician ideology variables are also linked. Liberal political ideology is positively correlated with higher obligation to treat stigmatized patients ($r = .257$, $p < .001$).

CONCLUDING REMARKS

The descriptive findings from this study are generally consistent with those of previous studies as reviewed in Chapters Two and Three. Female, minority, and foreign-born physicians in the 1990 national survey were significantly more likely than non-Hispanic, white, U.S. born male physicians to work in the less prestigious lower paying specialty of pediatrics and significantly less likely to work in the higher prestige, higher paying specialty of surgery. Other studies have found that female and minority physicians are much more likely than male and white physicians to practice in lower-paying primary care specialties (Altekruse and McDermott 1988; Babbott, Weaver, and Baldwin 1994); and that pediatrics has the highest female to male physician ratio (Langwell 1982; Bowman and Gross 1986; AMA 1992) while being the lowest paying medical specialty (Bobula 1980).

The 1990 survey found that all three groups of marginal physicians were significantly more likely than dominant physicians to practice in institutional settings. This finding is consistent with that of other studies which indicate that women and minorities are overrepresented in salaried, institutionally-based positions (Adams and Bazzoli; Bowman and Gross 1986) and that foreign-born IMGs tend to fill residual positions in hospital settings (Stevens et al. 1978).

Findings from the present study indicate that all three groups of marginal physicians are more likely than dominant physicians to locate in areas with higher percentages of minority populations and that foreign-born and minority physicians, but not female physicians, are significantly more likely than dominant physicians to practice in locations with higher poverty rates. This finding is generally consistent with other studies indicating that young, minority physicians tend to be highly concentrated in urban areas (USDHHS 1993) and that foreign-born IMGs have traditionally filled vacancies in locations of high medical need, which include poor, urban minority communities (Stevens et al 1978). In contrast to the present study's findings, other studies (Adams and Bazzoli 1986; Hojat et al. 1990) have reported that female physicians are more likely to work in low-income neighborhoods than are male physicians.

The present study's finding that, in general, female, foreign-born, and minority physicians expressed greater political liberalism than dominant physicians is consistent with the findings of other researchers who have found greater political liberalism expressed by these groups in contrast to their respective colleagues (Colombotos and Kirchner 1986; Colombotos et al. 1977; Richard 1969).

Who Cares for Poor People

Table 5.9 Weighted Correlation Matrix of Major Study Variables

PMED (hi=hi % Medicaid patients)	PMED	GENDER	RACE	BIRTHP
GENDER (hi=female)	.171**			
RACE (hi=minority)	.212**	.147**		
BIRTHP (hi=foreign birthplace)	.149**	.116**	.645**	
MEDSCHL (hi=foreign med school)	.133**	.069	.536**	.766**
BOARDC (hi=not board-certified)	.136**	.054	.167**	.167**
PEDS (hi=pediatric specialty)	.191**	.166**	.046	.031
PRACSET (hi=institutional setting)	.367**	.222**	.095*	.022
MINORITY (hi=hi minority location)	.308**	.081	.263**	.151**
POVERTY (hi=hi poverty location)	.340**	.032	.129**	.061
POLIT ID (hi=liberal pol ideology)	.085+	.146**	.064	.052
OBTREAT (hi=obligation to treat)	.216**	.131**	125**	.159**

+ indicates the correlation is significant at the $p \leq .05$ level.
*   indicates the correlation is significant at the $p \leq .01$ level.
** indicates the correlation is significant at the $p \leq .001$ level.

Table 5.9 Weighted Correlation Matrix of Major Study Variables
(continued)

MEDSCHL (hi=IMG)	MEDSCHL	BOARDC	PEDS	PRACSET
BOARDC (hi=not board-certified)	.228**			
PEDS (hi=pediatric specialty)	.038	-.099*		
PRACSET (hi=institutional setting)	.016	.063	.075	
MINORITY (hi=hi minority location)	.101*	-.010	.068	.281**
POVERTY (hi=hi poverty location)	.013	-.030	.035	.262**
POLIT ID (hi=liberal pol ideology)	.019	-.020	.059	.190**
OBTREAT (hi=obligation to treat)	.133**	-.010	.184**	.176**

	MINORITY	POVERTY	POLIT ID
POVERTY (hi=hi poverty location)	.671**		
POLIT ID (hi=liberal pol ideology)	.102*	.025	
OBTREAT (hi=obligation to treat)	.093*	.059	.257**

* indicates the correlation is significant at the $p \leq .01$ level.

** indicates the correlation is significant at the $p \leq .001$ level.

VI

Physician Participation in Medicaid

Most physicians surveyed participated in Medicaid; that is, 84 percent of physicians reported that at least one percent of their patient population were Medicaid recipients (See Table 6.1). Wide variation existed, however, in the extent of their participation. Most physicians treated a small percentage of Medicaid patients in their practices, while a small number of physicians treated relatively large percentages of Medicaid patients. Approximately 73 percent of all physicians (including physicians who had no Medicaid patients) reported that less than 20 percent of their patient population were Medicaid recipients, while approximately nine percent of physicians reported that 50 percent or more of their clientele were Medicaid patients.

The average Medicaid caseload of physicians surveyed was approximately 15 percent; however, pediatricians were notably different from the other specialty groups. Pediatricians reported a mean of 24.5 percent of their patient population on Medicaid compared to 13.1 percent reported by all other physicians in the study (p < .001). The overrepresentation of pediatricians among those physicians reporting higher Medicaid patient caseloads reflects the fact that roughly 46 percent of eligible Medicaid beneficiaries in 1990 were children (USDHHS 1993).

Sixteen percent of the physician respondents (N=143 / 880) did not participate in Medicaid. (Among pediatricians, reported non-participation was 15 percent). Non-participants were evenly spread across institutional and office-based settings. Earlier studies of office-based physicians report

Table 6.1 Medicaid Participation by Physicians[1,2]

Medicaid patients as a % of all patients in physician' s practice	(N=880)	% of physicians participating[3]
None	143	16
1 to 9	317	36
10 to 19	186	21
20 to 29	80	9
30 to 39	58	7
40 to 49	15	2
50 to 59	31	4
60 to 69	16	2
70 to 79	10	1
80 to 89	15	2
90 to 100	9	1

[1] Response to the question: "About what percentage of your
    patients are covered by Medicaid?"
[2] All figures are weighted.
[3] Percentages add up to more than 100% due to rounding.

somewhat higher percentages of non-participation in Medicaid. Sloan et al. (1978) found that 23 percent of a national sample of office-based primary care physicians surveyed in 1976 did not participate in Medicaid. Using data from the same study, Mitchell (1983) found that 19 percent of medical and surgical specialists did not participate in Medicaid. Longitudinal studies of office-based pediatricians have reported increasing non-participation in Medicaid between 1978 and 1989. Perloff et al.' s (1987) study of pediatricians in 13 states found that 15 percent of office-based pediatricians in 1978, and 18 percent of pediatricians in 1983, did not participate in Medicaid. In a follow-up study, Yudkowsky, Cartland, and Flint (1990) found that 23 percent of office-based pediatricians in 1989 did not participate in Medicaid.

Since previous studies have not examined comparable samples of physicians to this study, the slight differences found in Medicaid participation are somewhat difficult to interpret; nevertheless, data from this study suggest that the vast majority of physicians see some Medicaid patients.

As noted in Chapter Four, previous research indicates that physicians tend to overestimate their participation in Medicaid in surveys based on self-report. These self-reports, however, are highly correlated with Medicaid participation as measured by office encounter data (Kletke et al. 1985). Furthermore, Kletke et al. (1985) showed that relationships between the independent variables and the two measures of Medicaid participation are approximately the same in regression analyses. It is therefore reasonable to conclude that, although physicians' self-reports may overstate Medicaid participation, this measure is a reliable dependent variable for further analyses.

RELATIONSHIPS BETWEEN THE INDEPENDENT AND DEPENDENT VARIABLES

All of the independent variables discussed—female gender, minority race/ethnicity, foreign birthplace, IMG status, no board certification, pediatric specialty, institutional setting, percent poverty and minority population of office location, political liberalism, and obligation to treat—are significantly related to extent of physicians' Medicaid participation (Table 6.2). Female, minority, and foreign-born physicians reported significantly higher average mean totals of patient population on Medicaid compared to their physician counterparts. International medical graduates and physicians who were not board-certified were overrepresented among physicians with higher Medicaid caseloads.

TABLE 6.2 Extent of Physician Medicaid Participation
by Categorical Variables[1]

Independent Variable	N	Mean % of Physician's Patient Population Covered by Medicaid
1. Gender		
Male	759	13.1
Female	119	22.9***
2. Race/Ethnicity		
White, non-Hispanic	700	12.5
Minority	162	23.2***
3. Birthplace		
U.S.	692	13.1
Foreign	172	20.4***
4. Medical Training		
USMG	692	13.1
IMG	187	19.4***
5. Board Certified		
Yes	662	12.9
No	216	19.1***
6. Medical Specialty		
All Other	774	13.1
Pediatrics	105	24.5***
7. Practice Setting		
Solo/Groups	729	11.3
Institutional	148	30.3***

[1] All figures are weighted.
*** $p \leq .001$

Correlations between extent of physician Medicaid participation and continuous variables in the study (see Table 5.9—Correlation Matrix) indicate that: liberal political ideology showed a very small positive correlation (r = .08, p < .05), and obligation to treat stigmatized patients a larger correlation (r = .22, p < .001) with greater Medicaid participation. Both percent minority population (r = .31, p < .001) and poverty rate (r = .34, p < .001) of physician practice location demonstrated relatively high positive correlations with greater physician participation in Medicaid.

The overrepresentation of IMGs and physicians without board certification among those with higher Medicaid caseloads is consistent with other physician surveys (Sloan et al. 1978; Mitchell and Cromwell 1980; Mitchell 1983; Fairbrother et al. 1995) as noted in Chapter Two. Numerous studies have also demonstrated that Medicaid patients are much more likely than other patients to obtain health care in institutional settings, particularly in states that offer less reimbursement relative to fee-for-service and Medicare payments (PPRC 1991).

RELATIONSHIP OF MULTIPLE MARGINAL STATUSES TO MEDICAID PARTICIPATION

Physicians were then grouped by the number of marginal statuses they possessed in order to compare the extent of their participation in Medicaid. Table 6.3 shows that the physicians with more marginal social statuses reported greater percentages of Medicaid patients in their practices compared to those with fewer marginal social statuses. Physicians with no marginal social statuses (white, male, and U.S. born), approximately 67 percent of all physicians surveyed, reported an average of 12 percent of their patient population on Medicaid. Physicians with three marginal statuses (minority, female, and foreign-born), less than four percent of all physicians surveyed, reported an average of 27 percent of their patient population on Medicaid.

Table 6.3   Number of Physician Marginal Statuses by Physician
             Participation in Medicaid[1]

NUMBER OF MARGINAL STATUSES	N	Mean % of Patients on Medicaid
1. None	576	12
2. One	147	16*
3. Two	104	24**
4 Three	32	27**

[1] All figures are weighted.

* $p \leq .05$ (Group 2 vs. Group 1)

** $p \leq .01$ (Group 3 vs. Group 2) (Group 4 vs. Group 2)

REGRESSION ANALYSIS

Multiple regression analyses were used to determine the influence of each independent variable on the dependent variable "percent of physician's patient population on Medicaid" while controlling for other independent variables. Initial regression models showed significant lack of fit to the assumption of normal error distribution. Subsequent regression diagnostics revealed that the dependent variable was skewed toward extreme values. A log-transformation of the dependent variable resolved the problem of non-normal error distribution and is used for the following analyses.

Table 6.4 presents findings of a regression analysis using "percent of physician's patient population on Medicaid" as the dependent variable. Study phase and mode of interview, as noted in Chapter Four, were entered as co-variates. The values of the standardized and unstandardized coefficients indicate that no board certification, pediatric specialty, institutional practice setting, high poverty practice location, and obligation

Table 6.4 Model I - Multiple Regression of "Percentage of Patients on Medicaid" on Other Factors[1,2]

Independent Variable	B	SE B	Beta
Female Gender	-0.121	0.126	-0.032
Minority Race/ Ethnicity	0.236	0.142	0.071+
Foreign-born	0.180+	0.176	0.056
International Medical Graduate	-0.235	0.157	-0.075
No Board Certification	0.276	0.098	0.093**
Pediatric Specialty	0.349	0.132	0.087**
Institutional Setting	0.470+	0.116	0.140***
High Minority Area Practice Location	-0.416	0.229	-0.081+
High Poverty Area Practice Location	3.916	0.494	0.344***
Liberal Political Ideology	0.058	0.045	0.042
Professional Obligation to Treat	0.227	0.055	0.143***
R^2 (Adjusted) = .190			$F=15.74$***

[1]All figures are weighted.
[2]Controlled for phase and mode of interview
+ $p \leq .10$
* $p \leq .05$
** $p \leq .01$
*** $p \leq .001$

to treat exert the greatest impact on "percent Medicaid patient population." All of these variables are significant at the p≤ .01 level. The minority racial/ethnic status of physicians also demonstrates statistically significant effects on "percent Medicaid patient population" at the p≤ .10 level. Female gender, foreign birthplace, international medical graduate status, and high minority practice location do not exert independent effects on "percent Medicaid patient population." The effect of liberal political ideology is not statistically significant.

As noted earlier, pediatricians were significantly more likely than all other specialists to be board-certified in one or more medical specialties. Thus, the positive relationship between pediatric specialty and board certification actually suppresses the relationship between no board certification and higher Medicaid caseloads.

The adjusted R^2 for the model in Table 6.4 indicates that the independent variables explain 19 percent of the variation in the dependent variable, physician participation in Medicaid. This model is statistically significant at the $p \leq .001$ level.

Findings in Table 6.4 also indicate that several variables included in the regression model do not contribute significantly to the R^2 in the model. In order to construct a more parsimonious model, the following variables were excluded because their standardized Beta coefficients were not significant (at $p > .10$): female gender, foreign-born status, IMG status, and liberal political ideology. Minority practice location was excluded from this regression equation because of its high positive correlation with poverty practice location.

Table 6.5 presents the results of a reduced model that includes the variables minority race/ethnicity, no board certification, pediatric specialty, institutional setting, high poverty practice location, and high professional obligation to treat stigmatized patients. The adjusted R^2 for the model in Table 6.5 indicates that the independent variables explain approximately the same amount of variation in the dependent variable (19 percent) as the larger model in Table 6.4. The reduced model is statistically significant at the $p \leq .001$ level.

Table 6.5 Model II - Multiple Regression of "Percentage of Patients on Medicaid" on Other Factors[1,2]

Independent Variable	B	SE B	Beta
Minority Race/ Ethnicity	0.171	0.108	0.051
No Board Certification	0.25	0.096	0.084**
Pediatric Specialty	0.315	0.131	0.078*
Institutional Setting	0.447	0.112	0.133***
High Poverty Area Practice Location	3.375	0.38	0.296***
Professional Obligation to Treat	0.239	0.053	0.151***
R^2 (Adjusted) = .188		F=24.55***	

[1]All figures are weighted.
[2]Controlled for phase and mode of interview
* $p \leq .05$
** $p \leq .01$
*** $p \leq .001$

EFFECTS ANALYSIS

In order to assess the relative effects of Social Marginality, Professional Marginality, and Ideology in explaining variation in physicians' Medicaid participation, the variables were grouped in a temporal order as follows :

1. *Social Marginality:*   Minority race/ethnicity

2. *Professional Marginality*:   No board certification
                                        Institutional practice
                                        Pediatric specialty
                                        Poverty practice location

3. *Ideology:*   High obligation to treat
                                        treat stigmatized patients

These three groups of variables were introduced in separate steps to assess their unique contribution to the coefficient of multiple determination R^2. The order of entry was then changed in order to separate the direct, indirect, and spurious effects of each set of variables (Davis 1985: 44-48). Tables 6.6 through 6.9 present an effects analysis which summarize the findings.

DISCUSSION OF THE EFFECTS ANALYSIS

Table 6.6 indicates that Social Marginality (minority race/ethnicity) acts on Medicaid participation largely indirectly through Professional Marginality and Ideology, the "intervening" variables. (There are no "prior" variables.) The direct effect of Social Marginality accounts for only about one percent of the total variation in the dependent variable (.002 / .188), while the indirect effect accounts for approximately nine percent of the total variation in the dependent variable (.017 / .188) in the model.

Table 6.6 Effects Analysis—Social Marginality (minority race/
ethnicity)

| Effect | Controlling | | |
	All Priors	All Intervening	Data
A. Total (Change in R^2)	no	no	+.019
B. Causal	yes	no	+.019
C. Direct	yes	yes	+.002
D. (A - B) = spurious due to priors			0
E. (B - C) = indirect due to intervenors			+.017
Causal:			
direct effect	.002	11%	
indirect effects	.017	89%	
	0	0	spurious
	.019	100%	

Table 6.7 Effects Analysis—Professional Marginality (no board
certification, Pediatrics, institutional setting, poverty location)

| Effect | Controlling | | |
	All Priors	All Intervening	Data
A. Total (Change in R^2)	no	no	+.169
B. Causal	yes	no	+.153
C. Direct	yes	yes	+.136
D. (A - B) = spurious due to priors			+.016
E. (B - C) = indirect due to intervenors			+.017
Causal:			
direct effect	.136	80%	
indirect effects	.017	10%	
	.016	9%	spurious
	.169	100%	

Table 6.8 Effects Analysis—Ideology (obligation to treat)

Effect	All Priors	All Intervening	Data
	Controlling		
A. Total (Change in R^2)	no	no	+.046
B. Causal	yes	no	+.022
C. Direct	yes	yes	+.022
D. (A - B) = spurious due to priors			+.024
E. (B - C) = indirect due to intervenors			0
Causal:			
direct effect	.022	49%	
indirect effect	0	0	
	.024	52%	spurious
	.046	100%	

Table 6.9 Decomposition of the Indirect Effects of Social Marginality
           on the Dependent Variable

A. Total effects of Social Marginality (Change in R^2)		+.019
B. Social Marginality adjusted for Ideology		+.013
C. (A - B) = indirect effect through Ideology		+.006
D. Total indirect effect of Social Marginality		+.017
E. (D - C) = indirect effect through		+.011
Professional Marginality		
Indirect effects through Ideology	.006	35%
Indirect effects through Professional Marginality	.011	65%
Total indirect effects	.017	100%

Table 6.9 shows the decomposition of the indirect effects of Social Marginality indicating that it operates largely through Professional Marginality (65 percent of the total indirect effect of Social Marginality) and, to a lesser extent, through Ideology (35 percent of the total indirect effect of Social Marginality).

In other words, findings from this analysis suggest that it is not the marginal social status of minority race/ethnicity per se that accounts for physicians' participation in Medicaid. Rather, physicians' marginal status (minority race/ethnicity) appears to affect their Medicaid caseloads because minority physicians are overrepresented among those with marginal professional statuses and characteristics, and, to a lesser extent, among those physicians expressing a greater obligation to treat stigmatized patients.

Table 6.7 presents an effects analysis of Professional Marginality variables taking into consideration "prior" (social marginality) and "intervening" (physician ideology) variables. The direct effects of the Professional Marginality variables contribute about 72 percent (.136 / .188) of the variation in the dependent variable; indirectly, through Ideology, they contribute about nine percent (.017 /.188) of the variation in the dependent variable. Through direct and indirect effects, these variables account for about 81 percent (.153 /.188) of the association in the model. Professional Marginality, then, explains most of the variation in physicians' Medicaid participation .

Table 6.8 presents an effects analysis of the Professional Ideology variable taking into consideration "prior" (social marginality and professional marginality) variables. (There are no "intervening" variables.) The direct effects of physician Ideology (that is, obligation to treat stigmatized patients) accounts for approximately 12 percent (.022 / .188) of the change in variation of the dependent variable. Thus, Ideology appears to have small direct effects on physician participation in Medicaid.

CONCLUSION

The social status of physicians (minority race/ethnicity) has small effects on participation in Medicaid and those effects are explained mainly indirectly through its relationship to professional ideology and professional statuses and characteristics. Professional statuses (pediatric specialty, no board certification) and characteristics (institutional practice setting, poverty location of physician practice) have the strongest effects on Medicaid participation and most of this effect is direct. Physicians' professional ideology (or obligation to treat stigmatized patients) has small but statistically significant effects on their participation in Medicaid.

DISCUSSION

As noted in Chapter Two, data for this study were collected at one point in time; as such, causal relationships among all the variables studied cannot be established conclusively. The findings of this study, however, taken together with the conceptual framework and empirical research reviewed in Chapter Three suggest some areas for future research.

Findings from this study are consistent with other studies suggesting that female, minority, and foreign-born and foreign-educated physicians are most likely to care for Medicaid patients. This study has argued that structural constraints on these physicians, who are marginal to the profession, operate to push them into a variety of less desirable practice settings and locations as well as into less prestigious specialties. As noted in Chapter Three, this phenomenon occurs through a variety of social mechanisms, including sponsorship and boycott, as well as through tangible factors such as fewer financial resources and loan indebtedness (particularly for racial and ethnic minorities), inflexible schedules (for women, especially, who tend to have numerous personal as well as professional demands on their time), and barriers to licensing for IMGs.

Female, minority, and foreign-born physicians in this study expressed a greater obligation to treat stigmatized patients compared to white, male, U.S. born physicians. Findings from this analysis also suggest that, to a lesser extent, marginal physicians' obligation to treat stigmatized patients, also accounts for the higher percentages of Medicaid patients in their practices. Marginal physicians' political ideology, as measured by political liberalism, appears to have no influence on their acceptance of Medicaid patients.

This study was not able to adequately investigate the overlapping statuses of female gender, minority race and ethnicity, and foreign-birth because of small sample sizes within these subcategories. Findings do point out, however, that the majority of minority group physicians are foreign-born and foreign-educated and that women are overrepresented within this group of physicians. This finding suggests that one group of physicians—female, minority, foreign-born and foreign-educated— is the most likely group to provide medical care to Medicaid patients.

VII

Summary and Policy Implications

Chapter Six found that physicians with marginal social statuses were more likely than those with no marginal statuses to provide care to greater numbers of Medicaid patients. Further analysis showed that most of the effect of social status on Medicaid participation is explained mostly through the greater likelihood that individuals with marginal social statuses also possess marginal professional statuses and characteristics. Physicians' professional ideology also appears to have a small direct effect, while their political ideology appears to have no effect, on their participation in Medicaid.

In this chapter I first discuss findings from this study in relation to the concepts of social marginality, professional marginality, and the socialization of marginal groups within the medical profession as well as directions for future research. Secondly, I address some implications of these findings for physician participation in Medicaid in the 1990s.

MARGINALITY IN THE MEDICAL PROFESSION

The Accumulation of Marginality

As defined in Chapter Two and described in Chapter Three, marginality results from a process of formal or informal discrimination and barriers to advancement in a profession. Through a series of social processes elaborated upon in Chapter Three, those individuals with less desirable social statuses find that opportunities for advancement within the profession are limited. The process is cumulative, so that the person of marginal social status is viewed as less deserving and consequently given fewer opportunities. This is the reverse side of the Matthew effect which posits that those who are viewed as more deserving, accumulate more opportunities and rewards. Marginality in the medical profession results from a gradual "accumulation" of marginal statuses. This process is best illustrated by the experience of foreign-born physicians.

Foreign-born physicians, as outsiders in a dominant culture, are at a social disadvantage. They become more disadvantaged and even less desirable if they have graduated from a medical school outside of the U.S. since foreign medical schools are generally perceived as providing a lesser educational experience (Foreman 1990). U.S. medical schools also provide important socializing experiences in becoming an American physician. Stevens et al. (1978) pointed out that foreign-born international medical graduates may be perceived as less competent because of cultural "deficiencies" rather than lack of skill or knowledge.

As noted in Chapter Three, career success, to a large extent, depends on sponsorship by powerful mentors, socialization into the profession, and prestige of internship hospital. Because they are perceived as less competent, IMGs may be given fewer opportunities to be mentored by powerful sponsors and to gain or demonstrate their competency. Mick (1987) found that IMGs were more likely than USMGs to enter into lower prestige hospitals and lower prestige medical practices in less desirable locations.

The literature has not established the reasons why IMGs are less likely than USMGs to be board-certified, but it is worth noting that large numbers of IMGs enter the U.S. for training programs (Tan 1977; Mick and Lee 1997). Board certification in a specialty involves a series of complex requirements which include the successful completion of an approved residency training program and examinations (AMA 1987). If an IMG has not completed an approved training program, she or he may not be eligible for specialty board certification. Financial barriers to a prolonged certification process as well as language barriers may be additional reasons why IMGs are significantly less likely to become board-certified.

Thus, physicians with marginal social statuses, in establishing themselves professionally, tend to accumulate marginal professional statuses and characteristics that build upon one other. Their decreasing opportunities and the consequent "accumulation of marginality" influences the likelihood that they will locate in less desirable (usually low-income) areas and thereby take larger numbers of Medicaid patients as a percentage of their total patient population.[1]

Female and minority physicians are concentrated in the primary care specialties, especially pediatrics, one of the lower prestige, lower paying specialties. They are also underrepresented in the surgical specialties, which include the highest prestige and highest income specialties. Female and minority physicians are also overrepresented in institutional practice settings which are significantly more likely than solo or group practices to be located in high poverty, high minority population areas.

Bergner (1970) has pointed out that selection into professional statuses works in two ways: first, the selection of preferred physicians by institutions; and secondly, the selection by individual physicians into particular institutions or locations. A similar process takes place in the selection of specialty and practice setting. Davidson's (1979) and Lorber's (1984) studies suggest that individuals make choices in recognition of their limited options within the profession. In other words, marginal physicians choose specialties and practice settings with the (conscious or unconscious) knowledge that some specialties and practice settings are more hospitable and accommodating than others.

As elaborated in Chapter Three, it is quite plausibly the marginalization of individuals with less valued social statuses that explains the concentration of women and minorities in the lower prestige primary care specialties and institutional settings. Adams and Bazzoli (1986) have also pointed out that anticipated peer discrimination may prevent female and minority physicians from seeking positions in partnership and group practices.

Socialization of the Marginal Person

The phenomenon of marginality in the medical profession raises an obvious question: "How can marginal groups be incorporated into the mainstream of the medical profession?" Chapter Three highlighted the centrality of informal socialization experiences including sponsorship and colleague networks in the development of successful medical careers. Practically oriented proposals should be built around both formal and informal processes of support.

Rinke (1981b) has noted that interpersonal relationships are crucial to professional socialization. Intensive and extensive personal relationships with the professional staff as well as regular contact with colleagues are key to the development of a professional identity. The informal exchange of information within professional relationships provides the novice with analytic skills and insider knowledge regarding her or his performance within the power structure of medicine.

Hall (1946, 1948, 1949) and Lorber (1984) have highlighted the importance of sponsorship in physician groups. Through relationships with a sponsor, the novice gains skills and important insights into the practice of her/ his profession. Lorber concluded that women in male-dominated professions need the sponsorship of established members of inner circles to document their worth as colleagues. The same is true of other marginal groups in medicine. Physicians with less valued social statuses, whether female, minority race/ethnicity, or IMGs, need powerful sponsors to promote them as capable professionals within the colleague group.

Kanter (1977) has suggested that since sponsorship is a central facet of career building, organizations and professional groups could extend it to greater numbers of people by making it a formal part of a management system and rewarding established persons who mentor novices. Some medical schools have successfully experimented with formal mentorship programs for minority students (Peterson and Carlson 1992).

Proportional representation of women and minorities in medical school faculties provides powerful role models for marginal students. These physicians, subsequently, may advocate for the interests and viewpoints of marginal students who are on the periphery of the dominant medical school culture. One AAMC study of U.S. medical schools showed a positive association between the presence of minority faculty and the graduation rates of minority students (AAMC 1987).

Lorber (1984) has underscored the importance of colleague groups and networks in defusing auxiliary statuses (such as gender, race, and ethnicity) that hinder professional advancement. She argues that individually, the marginal person is vulnerable to all aspects of informal discrimination—relegation to sex-stereotyped work, minimizing of achievements, lack of visibility for promotion to positions of authority, and a target of criticism for either commitment to or neglect of family responsibilities. The marginal person who embarks on a career path isolated from others in her/his status group, is likely to ignore the subtle effects of informal discrimination on the job and is perceived as a troublemaker if she/he takes formal action against discriminatory practices. It is within colleague groups, however, that physicians with marginal statuses can effectively address formal and informal discriminatory practices.

Socialization and Ideology

Results in Chapters Five and Six showed that physicians with socially marginal statuses were more likely than dominant physicians to express liberal political ideology and greater obligation to treat stigmatized patients which, in turn, was positively correlated to greater percentages of Medicaid patients. The regression model in Chapter Six indicated that the small positive relationship between liberal political ideology and greater Medicaid participation was completely explained by the social and professional statuses of those physicians. Previous studies have also found more politically liberal attitudes among female (Colombotos and Kirchner 1986), African American (Richard 1969), and foreign-educated physicians (Colombotos et al. 1977) than among their respective physician counterparts.

Freidson (1970: 87-108) has argued that the immediate work environment exerts a more important influence on physicians' performance and attitudes than does early socialization. Colombotos and Kirchner (1986: 106-107) have suggested that socialization in the statuses of specialty and worksetting affects the attitudes of physicians more strongly than does their selection into a particular specialty and worksetting.

Findings from the present study indicate that among the professional characteristics and statuses, institutional worksetting and pediatric specialty are most strongly related to greater obligation to treat stigmatized patients (Table 5.9—Correlation Matrix).[2] It is quite plausible that physicians' greater obligation to treat stigmatized patients results from their professional socialization through institutional worksettings and pediatric specialty.

It is more difficult for physicians in institutional settings to refuse to provide care for patients compared with physicians in private practice. Freidson observes that workplace settings exert distinct influences on the provision of care. He notes that, historically, hospitals grew up separately from mainstream medical practice (Freidson 1970 : 110). Hospitals and other institutional settings, such as veterans hospitals and community health centers, have traditionally been places where the poor who lacked access to medical care could obtain appropriate care. Thus, it appears that the culture of institutional settings supports professional norms regarding physicians' obligation to treat all patients as well as their legal requirement to do so. A physician in an office setting can work alone and exercise more independent judgement than can a physician in an institutional setting who works as one member of a larger group of health care providers.

It is also plausible that pediatric specialty provides a distinctive socialization within the medical profession. Twentieth century American society places great emphasis on the protection of children as a vulnerable group in the population. Because becoming a pediatrician involves the care of children, it may also foster a greater sense of obligation to treat all vulnerable or stigmatized groups in the society.

Although the correlations between the three marginal social statuses and obligation to treat are highly significant in this study (Table 5.9—Correlation Matrix), the relationship of foreign birth and obligation to treat stigmatized patients is the strongest. Foreign-born physicians, whether naturalized citizens or not, are in a more precarious position in the U.S. than are native born physicians. They might feel, consciously or unconsciously, that their position in the U.S. is contingent upon their adherence to professional norms and legal requirements. This is particularly true since they are allowed into the U.S. for the specific task of practicing medicine. It is possible that foreign-born physicians may feel less secure in their professional positions and more constrained by ethical norms and legal requirements regarding treatment of patients.[3]

Physician Ideology

Findings from this study indicate that the association between physicians' political ideology and Medicaid participation, small to begin with, is completely explained by other variables in the model. Small positive effects between greater obligation to treat stigmatized patients and Medicaid participation indicate that, although physicians who express greater ethical obligation and feel legally required to care for stigmatized patients see more Medicaid patients, this accounts for a relatively small amount of the total variance in explaining physicians' participation in Medicaid.

It should be noted that the variables used to assess physician ideology in this study were somewhat inadequate. It is possible that additional measures of physicians' attitudes toward social welfare issues and care of the poor would have enhanced the relationship between ideology and Medicaid participation found in the model.

DIRECTIONS FOR FUTURE RESEARCH

This study relies on a broad literature to argue that marginal physicians' participation in Medicaid results from limitations on their professional opportunities. It is also possible, however, that it is the preferences of these groups of physicians that leads them to greater Medicaid participation. To answer this question, future research would, first, need to oversample groups of marginal physicians including those with multiple marginal social statuses. A longitudinal study design could compare physicians' expressed preferences regarding specialty and practice setting with later choices as well as the factors involved in their decisionmaking regarding specialty and practice setting. More detailed questions on political and professional ideology, particularly obligation to treat poor, minority, and underserved populations would add greater dimension to various factors related to physicians' preferences.

As noted in Chapter Three, advocates and policymakers have argued for a variety of policies to increase the numbers of minority physicians and to limit licensing restrictions for IMGs in the belief that these groups of physicians are most likely to care for poor Americans and underserved communities. Such proposals should also consider the fact that continued barriers in the medical profession are very likely restricting these groups of physicians to less desirable, less prestigious positions within medicine.

PHYSICIAN PARTICIPATION IN MEDICAID IN THE 1990s

The Impact of Medicaid Managed Care

Findings from the present study should be placed in the context of the dramatic changes occurring in Medicaid in the 1990s, namely, the restructuring of the program by managed care. Managed care will undoubtedly change the vocabulary and models that analysts employ to address physician participation in Medicaid. It erases the distinctions between traditionally "public" and "private" markets and strengthens the position of "third party payers" in the Medicaid debate (Silverstein 1997). Managed care may also weaken many of the relationships found in this study between professional statuses (international medical graduate, board certification, specialty) and characteristics (institutional setting, high minority population and poverty location) of physicians and their participation in Medicaid. In the following sections, I consider changes that might result from the widespread implementation of Medicaid managed care.

Board Certification of Physicians and Medicaid Participation

States vary in their implementation of Medicaid managed care programs (Sparer 1996; Gold, Sparer, and Chu 1996; Grogan 1997). Some states have high standards regarding the qualifications of Medicaid providers under managed care. Physicians in New York State, for example, must be either board-certified or eligible to qualify; if board eligible they must be certified within five years or less in a primary care specialty. Licensed nurse practitioners and physician assistants also qualify as primary care providers in Medicaid managed care arrangements (Kotelchuk 1994). If such requirements are adopted and strictly implemented by most states, non-board-certified and non-board eligible physicians will not be Medicaid providers, and board certification will no longer distinguish physicians on the basis of Medicaid caseload.

It is quite possible that other qualified, but lower paid primary care providers, such as nurse practitioners and physician assistants might replace physicians without board certification as Medicaid providers. This, in turn, may tend to displace socially marginal (female, minority, foreign-born) physicians and IMGs who disproportionately lack board certification.

Physician Specialty Patterns and Medicaid Managed Care

According to the AAMC, in 1995 there was a sharp increase in the number of medical students choosing primary care specialties such as family practice, internal medicine, and pediatrics and a decrease in popular specialties like radiology and anesthesiology (*New York Times* April 15, 1995). This trend continued through 1997 (Mick and Lee 1997) and follows a long term national trend away from primary care specialization (Colwill 1992). Some analysts attribute the shift to the impact of managed care plans which limit use of physician specialists. Retraining in primary care is one obvious option faced by underemployed specialists. In the long term, the implementation of managed care will probably increase the ratio of primary care to specialist physicians.

Although Adams and Bazzoli (1986) noted a possible trend toward increased specialization among white females and male minorities (but not among minority females), it is doubtful that this trend will continue if Medicaid managed care reduces the specialist to primary care physician ratio. Decreases in student financial support (*New York Times* June 6, 1995) and the movement away from affirmative action initiatives (*New York Times* January 25, 1995) in education nationwide make it even more unlikely that lower income students (who include more women and minorities) will be able to afford lengthy subspecialty training programs.

Physician Practice Setting and Medicaid Participation

One of the main objectives of managed care is to decrease costs by shifting the site of care from high cost emergency departments and outpatient clinics to less expensive office-based care and Health Maintenance Organizations (HMOs). Traditionally, institutional settings such as community health centers and hospital outpatient clinics have been an important site of care for Medicaid patients. Many such institutions, referred to as "safety-net providers," are newcomers in the managed care market and, consequently, have lost some of their traditional Medicaid patient base and revenues to managed care plans. Some institutions have created their own managed care plans or act as contractual providers within managed care plan networks and, as such, are continuing to provide services through Medicaid (Perloff 1996). Emergency department use by Medicaid patients, however, will most certainly decline if managed care delivers on its promises of better continuity of care.

Relationship Between High Minority and High Poverty Practice Locations and Medicaid Participation

There is no evidence to suggest that Medicaid managed care will radically restructure physicians' practice locations or in any way address the geographic maldistribution of physicians (Perloff 1996: 191-92; Gold, Sparer, and Chu 1996: 163; Sparer 1997: 805). Assuming that the present geographic distribution of physicians remains unchanged, managed care will probably enlarge the geographic area in which Medicaid patients obtain primary care. Because there are severe shortages of primary care physicians in low-income areas, Medicaid managed care will probably force patients to travel over greater distances to see primary care providers in managed care arrangements and prevent them from going to more convenient sites such as emergency departments or outpatient clinics. Lack of convenient sites for care may result in missed appointments, and consequently inadequate preventive care for many poor Americans.

Physicians outside of poverty areas, who have not cared for Medicaid patients, may be willing to see them under managed care arrangements. As Grogan (1997) points out, however, such assumptions may be naive given the historical experience of low physician participation in Medicaid. Anecdotal evidence from Connecticut indicates that Medicaid recipients in Blue Cross/Blue Shield do not have access to all providers in the commercial network (1997: 837).

POLICIES TO INCREASE PHYSICIANS IN POOR COMMUNITIES

The National Health Service Corps and Community Health Centers

As discussed in Chapter Two, severe shortages of physicians in low-income areas may decrease poor Americans ability to obtain appropriate, continuous medical care (Fossett and Peterson 1989; Fossett et al. 1990). A successful strategy to increase the physician work force in poor communities has been the development of the National Health Service Corps (NHSC). It is the largest source of medical school funding for physicians providing primary care in underserved[4] communities, many of which include disproportionate numbers of Medicaid patients.

Congress first authorized scholarships in 1972 for health professionals in return for a minimum of two years service in designated communities. NHSC was virtually defunded in the 1980s and then refunded in the early 1990s. The NHSC has also been highly successful in retaining providers in their site beyond their original service obligations, from 39 percent in 1991 to 64 percent in 1996 (U.S. Health Resources & Services Administration. April 1998. *Bureau of Primary Health Care Fact Sheet*).

Federally funded community health centers, a major provider of primary care to Medicaid patients and others in low-income communities since the mid-sixties, have been staffed by NHSC physicians. In the mid-eighties, NHSC physicians accounted for about fifty percent of community health clinics in the U.S. Drastic cuts in scholarships for NHSC physicians in the 1980s, however, resulted in a 25 percent physician shortage (800 unfilled slots) in federally-funded community health centers by the early-nineties (Sparer 1997: 796-97). Community health centers (CHCs) were found to be highly successful in increasing access to ambulatory health services, and in decreasing in-patient and emergency department usage among residents of low-income and minority communities in a comprehensive review of available utilization data (Freeman et al. 1982). Advocates argue that, as community-based institutions, CHCs provide essential, appropriate services to underserved communities (Gardner 1993; Blumenthal, Lukomnik, and Hawkins 1993).

Congressional appropriations supporting community health centers have increased in the 1990s. A new category of federally-qualified health centers where Medicaid reimburses services at full cost has been created (Kotelchuck 1994: 30-31). Community health centers and other hospital-linked clinics offer a reasonable, hopeful alternative for health care services to low-income communities. Schauffler and Wolin (1996) point out, however, that CHCs are particularly vulnerable in a managed care environment if not given governmental funding and safeguards, infrastructure support, and technical assistance and training.

Primary Care Career Pathways

Some advocates of primary care for underserved communities identify minority students as being especially well suited for roles as primary care providers in low-income communities. Presenters at the 1990 Second HRSA Primary Care Conference, for example, proposed an "urban health education center" (UHEC) whose specific focus would be the creation of a "primary care career pathway" for disadvantaged and minority students. In the UHEC, minority students would be tracked into intensive primary care career training programs (USDHHS 1990b: 147-182).

Such proposals are laudable to the extent that they attempt to address the health care needs of underserved areas; however, in linking the twin concerns of minority representation in medicine and primary care medicine for underserved communities, they risk situating lower income and underrepresented minority physicians into less prestigious and less desirable positions within the medical profession. Targeting lower income and underrepresented minority students for scholarships in primary care medicine effectively competes with the choice to pursue more technical specialty training and research tracks within medicine.

A more fruitful approach to both problems—too few students pursuing careers in primary care and low proportionate underrepresented minority representation in medicine—would be first, to retain proposed minority recruitment programs, which provide counseling and educational support programs at the undergraduate level for medical careers, without steering these students into primary care medicine per se; and secondly, to develop more and better primary care specialty training programs within medical schools. Tracking minority students into primary care medicine will only reinforce the stratification of the U.S. medical profession by race/ethnicity and gender.

CONCLUDING REMARKS

This study has attempted to elucidate the social processes of marginality in the American medical profession and to explain the relationship between marginal physicians and the medical care of poor Americans. Women, minorities, and IMGs have historically been marginal groups in American medicine and, as a result, have had fewer opportunities and more barriers to career satisfaction and success. Several promising remedies to overcome marginalization in the medical profession were discussed. These remedies include a broad mix of individual, small group, and formal and informal systems to achieve full integration of the U.S. medical profession.

While women comprise an increasingly larger proportion of physicians in the United States today, underrepresented racial and ethnic minorities do not. According to the USDHHS, African American and Hispanic physicians each comprised less than six percent of medical school graduates in 1991-1992. The size of the African American and Latino population in the U.S. is increasing at a faster rate than the rest of the population. By 2020, almost 25 percent of the U.S. population will be African American or Latino (USDHHS 1993: 2). America's success as a nation in the twenty-first century depends on its ability to maximally develop and use the talents and skills of all groups in society.

NOTES

1. One exception to the notion that marginal statuses "accumulate" is the fact that pediatricians in this study were more likely to be board-certified than other specialists.

2. Path analyses, conducted in the preliminary phase of this dissertation, indicated that foreign birthplace, pediatric specialty, and institutional setting exerted independent effects upon obligation to treat.

3. A contrasting view of minority professionals' adherence to professional norms is provided by Carlin (1966). In a study of New York City lawyers and ethics, he showed that those who possess minority status in a profession are less likely than the majority to uphold professional norms.

4. As part of the HMO Act of 1973, an Index of Medical Underservice was developed with the intention of identifying "medically underserved" communities in the U.S. The index is based on four qualities listed in order of importance: the ratio of primary care physicians to total population; the infant mortality rate; the percentage of persons with incomes below the poverty level; and the percentage of the population 65 and older (USDHHS 1990b: 106-107).

Appendix I

Sample Design and Selection[1]

For sampling purposes, the study population was defined as follows:

Physicians – All non-Federal physicians in office based and hospital based practice (excluding residence and clinical fellows) who were included in the 1989 American Medical Association (AMA) Masterfile, whose primary specialties were classified as Family Practice, General Practice, Pediatrics, Obstetrics-Gynecology, Internal Medicine and associated subspecialties, General Surgery, or Other Surgical Specialties.

The sample of physicians was obtained through the use of a probability sample design which involved three basic geographic strata. The three geographic strata were defined as: New York City (consisting of the counties of Bronx, Kings, Queens, Manhattan and Richmond); San Francisco (consisting of San Francisco County) and the balance of the 50 United States and the District of Columbia.

For the geographic strata of New York City and San Francisco, lists of physicians were obtained from the American Medical Association. Inclusion in the geographic strata of New York City or San Francisco was based on either a county code identification from the AMA Masterfile.

The sample of physicians for the New York City and San Francisco strata was selected by applying a systematic random sampling procedure to the separate list of physicians within each of the two strata. Prior to selection, physicians were sorted by county (in the case of New York City) and specialty. The population consisted of 10,376 and 1,746 physicians in New York City and San Francisco respectively. Samples of size 224 and 192 physicians were selected from these two strata.

The sample of physicians for the balance of the U.S. was selected by a two stage sampling procedure. In the first stage, a sample of 25 states was selected from the 50 United States and the District of Columbia. Selection probabilities were proportional to a measure of size that computed as the average of the proportion of U.S. physicians in the state.

Prior to sample selection states were sorted on the basis of geographic region. All states with a measure of size 35214.0 were included in the sample with certainty. This resulted in the selection of 15 states. The total measure of size for these certainty states was 576,723. The remaining 35 states and the District of Columbia accounted for a combined measure of size equal to 423,278. From these, a total of 10 states were selected (based on probabilities proportional to their measure of size) using a skip interval of 28218.53 and a random start of 22106.39.

Within each of the 25 selected states, a list of physicians was obtained from the AMA. For the states of New York and California, the list excluded physicians who were classified in the New York City and San Francisco strata.

The list was sampled, using systematic random sampling in order to produce the final sample of physicians. In order to produce an equal probability of selection for physicians across the various states, the rate of sub-sampling within each state was determined so that the product of the first stage of sampling times the second (within state) stage was equal to a constant over all states. More specifically, the probability of selection for physicians within the ith selected state was equal to $P_{2i} = K/P_{1i}$, where P_{1i} denotes the probability of selection in stage one and K is a constant. Thus, the overall probability of selection for physicians in the it state is equal to $f_i = P_{1i} \times P_{2i} = P_{1i} \times (K/P_{1i}) = K$.

Prior to selection within state physicians were sorted by county and specialty within county. The following table shows the number of physicians within each of the 25 states selected in the first stage of sampling. The table also shows the first stage probability of selection for these 25 first stage units. Over the 25 states selected in the first stage of selection, the second stage of sampling resulted in the selection of 1,280 physicians.

MD Sub-sample

In October 1990, due to a low response rate, a sub-sample of 50% of the remaining MD cases was drawn. The sub-sample of physicians was selected by applying a simple random sampling procedure to the list of physicians who had not completed interviews as of October 12, 1990 and who, based on preliminary contact to date, were still believed to be eligible for the survey. Of these remaining 805 cases, 403 were chosen as part of the sub-sample.

---

[1]Excerpted from the description of the sample design and selection for physicians and nurses for Physicians, Nurses, and AIDS: Findings From A National Study (unpublished NORC memo, October 29, 1991)

Table of Physicians Selected for Survey Sample

STATE	DRs–AMA	PROB1	PROB2	DRs–TAKE
Arizona	3773	0.467281	0.010559	40
California	34470	1.	0.004934	170
Connecticut	4655	0.638764	0.007725	36
Washington,DC	1397	0.238885	0.020656	29
Florida	15175	1.	0.004934	75
Georgia	6126	0.696563	0.007084	43
Illinois	12540	1.	0.004934	62
Indiana	5013	0.672040	0.007342	37
Iowa	2269	0.427095	0.011553	26
Kentucky	3564	0.404131	0.012210	44
Louisiana	4448	0.485567	0.010162	45
Massachusetts	7958	1.	0.004934	39
Michigan	8284	1.	0.004934	41
Missouri	5090	0.709250	0.006957	35
New Jersey	10116	1.	0.004934	50
New York	14640	1.	0.004934	72
North Carolina	6482	0.775199	0.006365	41
Ohio	10757	1.	0.004934	53
Pennsylvania	13841	1.	0.004934	68
South Carolina	3057	0.345978	0.014262	44

Table of Physicians Selected for Survey Sample (Continued)

STATE	DRs–AMA	PROB1	PROB2	DRs–TAKE
Tennessee	5110	0.607543	0.008121	42
Texas	15647	1.	0.004934	77
Washington	5343	0.690928	0.007141	38
Wisconsin	5024	0.689936	0.007152	36
Wyoming	418	0.055070	0.089603	37

Total   1280

$K = 0.004934$

Appendix II

Study Measures

Gender
0.   Male
1.   Female

Race/Ethnicity
0.   White
- White, non-Hispanic

1.   Minority:
- Black, non-Hispanic
- Hispanic
- Filipino
- Other Asian or Pacific Islander
- Other

Country of Birth
0.   U.S.
1.   Other

Medical School
0.   U.S. Medical Graduate
1.   International Medical Graduate

Board Certification
0.   Board certified in one or more specialties
1.   No board certification

Medical Specialty

0.   Other
- Family/Group practice
- Internal Medicine
- Obstetrics/Gynecology
- Surgery

1.   Pediatrics

Practice Setting

0.   Solo_Group practice includes:
- Individual private practice
- Partnership with one other physician
- Private group practice
- HMOs if solo or group setting

1.   Institutionally-based includes:
- Hospital-based practice (inpatient, outpatient clinic, emergency room);
- Other institutionally based practice (including nursing home, company or industrial clinic, school clinic, neighborhood health center, etc.)

Political Ideology

"In your political thinking, do you consider yourself...very liberal, liberal, middle-of-the-road, conservative, or very conservative?"

RESPONSE CATEGORIES:
1.   Very conservative
2.   Conservative
3.   Middle-of-the-road
4.   Liberal
5.   Very liberal

Obligation To Treat Scale
Standarized Item Alpha = .93

T1.   Physicians in their office practice should be legally required to provide care

T2.   Attending physicians in the hospital should be legally required to provide care

T3.   Surgeons should be legally required to provide care

T4.   Registered nurses in the hospital should be legally required to provide care

T5.   It is professionally unethical for you to refuse to care

T6.   It is professionally unethical for physicians in their office practice to refuse to care

T7.   It is professionally unethical for attending physicians in the hospital to refuse to care

T8.   It is professionally unethical for surgeons to refuse to care

T9.   It is professionally unethical for registered nurses in the hospital to refuse to care

RESPONSE CATEGORIES:
1.   Disagree strongly
2.   Disagree somewhat
3.   Agree somewhat
4.   Agree strongly

Appendix III

Calculation of U.S. Census Variables[1]

1.   1990 U.S. Census Percent Minority Population of Zipcode Area
        computed from:

> 1.00 - ("Not of Hispanic Origin White" /
> "100 Percent Count of Persons")

2.   1990 U.S. Census Poverty Rate of Zipcode Area
        computed from:

> ("Ratio of Income in 1989 to Poverty Level"
> $\sum$ 0 through .99) / ("Universe of Persons for
> Whom Poverty Status is Determined")

---

[1] data obtained from the U.S. Department of Commerce, Economics and
Statistics Administration, Bureau of the Census (1994) *1990 Decennial
Census of Population and Housing* on CD-ROM, Washington, DC.

Appendix IV

Standardized Scale Construction[1]

Scale items were standardized for the Colombotos et al. study (1995). "Obligation to Treat" measures included a four-item "Legal Obligation to Treat" and a five-item "Ethical Obligation to Treat" scale. A standardized scale was constructed by standarizing each item, multiplying it by its associated factor score, and summing these products. When individual items in a scale were missing values, one of two procedures was followed. If fewer than half the items for a given respondent were missing values, a regression procedure, IMPUTE in STATA (Computing Resource Center, STATA Reference Manual, Release 2.1, Computer Resource Center, Santa monica CA: 1990) was used to assign missing values. If a respondent had half or more of the items in a scale missing, s/he was assigned a missing value for that scale.

---

[1]parts excerpted from Colombotos et al. (1993) *Physicians, Nurses, and AIDS: Findings from a National Study* Unpublished Final Report to AHCPR.

Bibliography

Acton, Jan Paul. 1976. "Demand for Health Care Among the Urban Poor, with Special Emphasis on the Role of Time." Pp. 165–208 in *The Role of Health Insurance in the Health Services Sector*, ed. R. Rosett. New York: National Bureau of Economic Research.

Adams, E. Kathleen, and Gloria J. Bazzoli. 1986. "Career Plans of Women and Minority Physicians: Implications for Health Manpower Policy." *Journal of the American Women's Medical Association* 41, no. 1: 17–20.

Altekruse, Joan M., and Suzanne W. McDermott. 1988. "Contemporary Concerns of Women in Medicine." Pp. 65–88 in *Feminism Within the Science and Health Professions: Overcoming Resistance*, ed. S.V. Rosser. Oxford: Pergamon Press.

American Medical Association (AMA). 1987. *Physician Characteristics and Distribution in the United States*. Chicago.

———. 1990. *Physician Characteristics and Distribution in the United States*. Chicago.

———. 1991. *Physician Characteristics and Distribution in the United States*. Chicago.

———. 1992. *Physician Characteristics and Distribution in the United States*. Chicago.

Anderson, Odin W., and Fremont J. Lyden. 1963. "Physicians, Third Party Payments, and Professional Prerogatives." *Journal of Health and Human Behavior* 4, no. 3: 195–99.

Association of American Medical Colleges (AAMC). 1987. *Differential Analysis of U.S. Medical Schools with High and Low Minority Graduation Rates: Final Report*. Washington, D.C.: Division of Medicine, Health Resources and Services Administration.

Babbott, David, DeWitt Baldwin, Charles D. Killian, and Sheila O'Leary Weaver. 1989. "Racial–Ethnic Background and Specialty Choice: A Study of U.S. Medical School Graduates." *Academic Medicine* 27, no. 9: 595–99.

Babbott, David, Sheila O. Weaver, and DeWitt C. Baldwin. 1994. "Primary Care by Desire or Default? Specialty Choices of Minority Graduates of U.S. Medical Schools." *Journal of the National Medical Association* 86, no. 7: 509–15.

Back, Kurt W., Robert E. Coker, Thomas G. Donnelly, and Bernard S. Phillips. 1958. "Public Health as a Career in Medicine: Secondary Choice Within a Profession." *American Sociological Review* 23, no. 5: 533–41.

Baker, David W., Carl D. Stevens, and Robert H. Brook. 1991. "Patients Who Leave a Public Hospital Emergency Department Without Being Seen by a Physician: Causes and Consequences." *Journal of the American Medical Association* 266, no. 8: 1085–90.

Bennett, Nancy M., and Katherine G. Nickerson. 1992. "Women in Academic Medicine: Perceived Obstacles to Advancement." *Journal of the American Women's Medical Association* 4: 115–18.

Bergner, Marilyn Ann. 1970. *Social Factors and Physicians' Choice of Physicians*. Ph.D. diss., Columbia University.

Bickel, Janet, and Phyllis R. Kopriva. 1993. "A Statistical Perspective on Gender in Medicine." *Journal of the American Women's Medical Association* 48, no. 5: 141–44.

Bindman, A.B., K. Grumbach, D. Keane, L. Rauch, and J.M. Luce. 1991. "Consequences of Queuing for Care at a Public Hospital Emergency Department." *Journal of the American Medical Association* 266: 1091–96.

Blackwell, James E. 1983. *Networking and Mentoring: A Study of Cross-Generational Experiences of Blacks in Graduate and Professional Schools*. Atlanta: Southern Education Foundation.

———. 1987. *Mainstreaming Outsiders: The Production of Black Professionals*. Dix Hills, N.Y.: General Hall, Inc.

Blum, Linda, and Vicki Smith. 1988. "Women's Mobility in the Corporation: A Critique of the Politics of Optimism." *Signs: Journal of Women in Culture and Society* 13 (spring): 528–45.

Blumenthal, Daniel S., Joanne E. Lukomnik, and Daniel R. Hawkins Jr. 1993. "A Proposal to Provide Care to the Uninsured through a Network of Community Health Centers." *Journal of Health Care for the Poor and Underserved* 4(3): 272–79.

Bobula, Joel D. 1980. "Work Patterns, Practice Characteristics, and Incomes of Male and Female Physicians." *Journal of Medical Education* 55 (October): 826–33.

Bowman, Marjorie, and Marcy Lynn Gross. 1986. "Overview of Research on Women in Medicine—Issues for Public Policymakers." *Public Health Reports* 101, no. 5: 513–21.

Brewer, Willis R., Merlin K. DuVal, and Gloria M. Davis. 1979. "Increasing Minority Recruitment to the Health Professions by Enlarging the Applicant Pool." *New England Journal of Medicine* 301, no. 2: 74–76.

Buono, Anthony F., and Judith B. Kamm. 1983. "Marginality and the Organizational Socialization of Female Managers." *Human Relations* 36, no. 12: 1125–40.

Cantor, Joel C., Erika L. Miles, Laurence C. Baker, and Dianne C. Barker. 1996. "Physician Serivce to the Underserved: Implications for Affirmative Action in Medical Education." *Inquiry* (summer): 167–80.

Carlin, Jerome Edward. 1966. *Lawyers' Ethics: A Survey of the New York City Bar.* New York: Russell Sage Foundation.

Cohen, Joel W. 1993. "Medicaid Physician Fees and Use of Physician and Hospital Services." *Inquiry* 30: 281–92.

Cole, Jonathan R. 1979. *Fair Science: Women in the Scientific Community.* New York: Free Press.

Cole, Stephen, Jonathan R. Cole, and G.A. Simon. 1981. "Chance and Consensus in Peer Review." *Science* 214: 881–86.

Colombotos, John. 1969. "Social Origins and Ideology of Physicians: A Study of the Effects of Early Socialization." *Journal of Health and Social Behavior* 10 (March): 16–29.

Colombotos, John, Catherine A. Charles, and Corinne Kirchner. 1977. "Physicians' Attitudes toward Political and Health Care Policy Issues in Cross–national Perspective: A Comparison of FMGs and USMGs." *Social Science and Medicine* 11, nos. 11–13: 603–9.

Colombotos, John, and Corinne Kirchner. 1986. *Physicians and Social Change.* New York: Oxford University Press.

Colombotos, John, Peter Messeri, Marianne McConnell, Jack Elinson, Donald Gemson, and Margaret Hynes. 1995. *Physicians, Nurses, and AIDS: Findings from a National Study.* Rockville, Md.: Agency for Health Care Policy and Research. Grant No.: 5R01 HS06359.

Colwill, Jack M. 1992. "Where Have All the Primary Care Applicants Gone?" *New England Journal of Medicine* 326, no. 6: 387–93.

Cornelius, Llewellyn. 1991. "Access to Medical Care for Black Americans with An Episode of Illness." *Journal of the National Medical Association* 83, no. 7: 617–26.

Crane, Diana. 1972. *Invisible Colleges: Diffusion of Knowledge in Scientific Communities.* Chicago: University of Chicago Press.

Cregler, Louis L. 1993. "Enrichment Programs to Create a Pipeline to Biomedical Science Careers." *Journal of the Association for Academic Minority Physicians* 4, no. 4: 127–31.

Cregler, Louis L., Luther T. Clark, and Edgar B. Jackson. 1994. "Careers in Academic Medicine and Clinical Practice for Minorities: Opportunities and Barriers." *Journal of the Association for Academic Minority Physicians* 5, no. 2: 68–73.

Davidson, Lynne R. 1979. "Choice by Constraint–The Selection and Function of Specialties Among Women Physicians–in–Training." *Journal of Health Politics, Policy and Law* 4, no. 2: 200–220.

Davidson, Stephen M. 1978. "Variations in State Medicaid Programs." *Journal of Health Politics, Policy and Law* 3: 54–70.

———. 1982. "Physician Participation in Medicaid." *Journal of Health Politics, Policy and Law* 6, no. 4: 703–17.

Davis, James A. 1985. *The Logic of Causal Order.* Beverly Hills: Sage Publications.

DeAngelis, Catherine D., and Michael E. Johns. 1995. "Promotion of Women in Academic Medicine: Shatter the Ceilings, Polish the Floors." *Journal of the American Medical Association* 273, no. 13: 1056–57.

Deming, W. Edwards. 1960. *Sample Design in Business Research*. New York: John Wiley & Sons.

Dublin, Thomas D. 1974. "Foreign Physicians: Their Impact on U.S. Health Care." *Science* 185, no. 4149: 407–14.

Dutton, Diana B. 1978. "Explaining the Low Use of Health Services by the Poor: Costs, Attitudes, or Delivery Systems?" *American Sociological Review* 43: 348–68.

Epps, Anna Cherrie, Mary T. Cureton–Russell, and Helen G. H. Kitzman. 1993. "Effective Strategies and Programs to Increase Minority Participation in the Health Professions for the 21st Century." *Journal of the Association for Academic Minority Physicians* 4, no.4: 116–26.

Epstein, Cynthia Fuchs. 1970. "Encountering the Male Establishment: Sex–status Limits on Women's Careers in the Professions." *American Journal of Sociology* 75, no. 6: 965–82.

———. 1971. *Woman's Place*. Berkeley: University of California Press.

Etzioni, Amitai. 1961. *A Comparative Analysis of Complex Organizations*. New York: The Free Press of Glencoe.

Fairbrother, Gerry, Kimberly A. DuMont, Stephen Friedman, and Katherine S. Lobach. 1995. "New York City Physicians Serving High Volumes of Medicaid Children: Who are They and How Do They Practice?" *Inquiry* 32 (fall): 345–52.

Foreman, Spencer. 1990. "Graduate Medical Education: Focus for Change." *Academic Medicine*: 77–84.

Fossett, James W., and John A. Peterson. 1989. "Physician Supply and Medicaid Participation." *Medical Care* 27, no. 4: 386–96.

Fossett, James W., Janet Perloff, John Peterson,and Phillip R. Kletke. 1990. "Medicaid in the Inner City: The Case of Maternity Care in Chicago." *The Milbank Quarterly* 68, no. 1: 111–41.

Fossett, James W., Chang H. Choi, and John A. Peterson. 1991. "Hospital Outpatient Services and Medicaid Patients Access to Care." *Medical Care* 29, no. 10: 964–76.

Fox, John G. and James M. Richards. 1977. "Physician Dominance and Location of Foreign and U.S.Trained Physicians." *Journal of Health and Social Behavior* 18 (December): 366–75.

Fredericks, Marcel A., Paul Mundy, and John Kosa. 1974. "Willingness to Serve: The Medical Profession and Poverty Programs." *Social Science and Medicine* 8, no. 1: 51–57.

Freeman, Howard E., K. Jill Kiecolt, and Harris M. Allen II. 1982. "Community Health Centers: An Initiative of Enduring Utility." *Health and Society* 60, no. 2: 245–67.

Freidson, Eliot. 1970. *Profession of Medicine: A Study of the Sociology of Applied Knowledge.* New York: Dodd, Mead, & Company.

Garber, Alan M. 1989. "Pursuing the Links Between Socioeconomic Factors and Health: Critique, Policy Implications, and Directions for Future Research." In *Pathways to Health,* eds. Bunker, Gomby, and Kehrer. Menlo Park, CA: The Henry J. Kaiser Family Foundation.

Gardner, Roland J. 1993. "National Health Care Reform and Community and Migrant Health Centers." *Journal of Health Care for the Poor and Underserved* 4(3): 268–71.

Garner, Dewey D., Winston C. Liao, and Thomas R. Sharpe. 1979. "Factors Affecting Physician Participation in a State Medicaid Program." *Medical Care* 17, no. 1: 43–58.

Gieryn, Thomas F., and Richard F. Hirsh. 1983. "Marginality and Innovation in Science." *Social Studies of Science* 13: 87–106.

Gold, Marcia, Michael Sparer, and Karyen Chu. 1996. "Medicaid Managed Care: Lessons From Five States." *Health Affairs* 15 (fall): 153–66.

Goldberg, Milton M. 1941. "A Qualification of the Marginal Man Theory." *American Sociological Review* 6, no. 1: 52–58.

Goldblatt, Arlene, Louis Wolf Goodman, Stephen S. Mick, and Rosemary Stevens. 1975. "Licensure, Competence, and Manpower Distribution." *New England Journal of Medicine* 292, no. 3: 137–41.

Golovensky, David I. 1952. "The Marginal Man Concept: An Analysis and Critique." *Social Forces* 30, no. 3: 333–39.

Goode, William J. 1957. "Community Within a Community: The Professions." *American Sociological Review* 22 : 195–200.

Green, Arnold W. 1947. "A Re–examination of the Marginal Man Concept." *Social Forces* 26, no. 1: 167–71.

Grogan, Colleen M. 1997. "The Medicaid Managed Care Policy Consensus for Welfare Recipients: A Reflection of Traditional Welfare Concerns." *Journal of Health Politics, Policy and Law* 22, no. 3: 815–38.

Groves, Robert M. 1989. *Survey Errors and Survey Costs.* New York: John Wiley & Sons.

Grumbach, Kevin, Dennis Keane, and Andrew Bindman. 1993. "Primary Care and Public Emergency Department Overcrowding." *American Journal of Public Health* 83, no. 3: 372–78.

Hadley, Jack. 1978. "An Econometric Analysis of Physician Participation in the Medicaid Program." *Working Paper.* 998–9 Washington, D.C.: The Urban Institute.

Hadley, Jack, Joel C. Cantor, Richard J. Willke, Judith Feder, and Alan B. Cohen. 1992. "Young Physicians Most and Least Likely to Have Second Thoughts about a Career in Medicine." *Academic Medicine* 67, no. 3: 180–90.

Hall, Oswald. 1946. "The Informal Organization of the Medical Profession." *Canadian Journal of Economics and Political Science* 12: 30–41.

———. 1948. "The Stages of a Medical Career." *American Journal of Sociology* 53, no. 5: 327–36.

———. 1949. "Types of Medical Careers." *The American Journal of Sociology* 55, no. 3: 243–53.

Hanson, Russell L. 1984. "Medicaid and the Politics of Redistribution." *American Journal of Political Science* 28: 313–19.

Harrington, William J., Eduardo Gotuzzo, Salvador Vial, et. al. 1991. "Estimating Impacts on Developing Countries of the Decrease in U.S. Training Opportunities for Foreign Medical Graduates." *Academic Medicine* 66 : 707–9.

Harris, Mary B., and Mary Ann Conley–Muth. 1981. "Sex Role Stereotypes and Medical Specialty Choice." *Journal of the American Medical Association* 36, no.8: 245–52.

Heins, Marilyn. 1985. "Update: Women in Medicine." *Journal of the American Medical Women's Association* 40, no.2: 43–50.

Hojat, Mohammadreza, Joseph S. Gonnella, J. Jon Veloski, and Shelly Moses. 1990. "Differences in Professional Activities, Perceptions of Professional Problems, and Practice Patterns between Men and Women Graduates of Jefferson Medical College." *Academic Medicine* 65, no. 12: 755–61.

Hughes, Everett C. 1971. *The Sociological Eye*. Chicago: Aldine Atherton.

Iglehart, John K. 1993. "The American Health Care System: Medicaid." *New England Journal of Medicine* 328, no. 12: 896–900.

Institute of Medicine (IOM). 1981. *Health Care in a Context of Civil Rights*. Washington, D.C.: National Academy Press.

———. 1996. *The Nation's Physician Workforce: Options for Balancing Supply and Requirements* Washington, D.C.: National Academy Press.

Intergovernmental Health Policy Project. 1983. *Recent and Proposed Changes in State Medicaid Programs: A Fifty State Survey*. (December). Washington D.C.: Intergovernmental Health Policy Project.

Jones, Michael W., and Bette Hamburger. 1976. "A Survey of Physician Participation in the Dissatisfaction with the Medi–Cal Program." *Western Journal of Medicine* (January): 75–83.

Kaiser Commission on the Future of Medicaid. 1997. *Medicaid Facts* (November). Washington, D.C.: The Kaiser Family Foundation.

Kandel, Denise B. 1960. *The Career Decisions of Medical Students: A Study in Occupational Recruitment and Occupational Choice*. Ph.D. diss., Columbia University.

Kanter, Rosabeth M. 1977. *Men and Women of the Corporation*. New York: Basic Books.

Kavaler, Florence. 1969. "Utopianism and Bare Knuckles in Public Health, IV. People, Providers and Payment Telling It How It Is." *American Journal of Public Health* 59, no. 5: 825–29.

Keith, Stephen N., Robert M. Bell, August G. Swanson, and Albert P. Williams. 1985. "Effects of Affirmative Action in Medical Schools: A Study of the Class of 1975." *New England Journal of Medicine* 313, no. 24:1519–25.

Keith, Stephen N. 1990. "Role of Minority Providers in Caring for the Underserved." *Journal of Health Care for the Poor and Underserved* 1, no. 1: 90–95.

Kirschstein, Ruth L. 1996. "Women Physicians—Good News and Bad News." *New England Journal of Medicine* 334, no.15: 982–83.

Kirsling, Robert A., and Mahendr S. Kochar. 1990. "Mentors in Graduate Medical Education at the Medical College of Wisconsin." *Academic Medicine* 65: 272–74.

Kletke, Phillip R., Stephen M. Davidson, Janet D. Perloff, Donald W. Schiff, and John P. Connelly. 1985. "The Extent of Physician Participation in Medicaid: A Comparison of Physician Estimates and Aggregated Patient Records." *Health Services Research* 20, no. 5 : 503–23.

Kletke, Phillip, and W. Marder, W. 1987. *The Geographic Distribution of Primary Care Physicians in Cook County, Illinois.* Chicago, Ill.: American Medical Association Center for Health Policy Research.

Komaromy, Miriam, Kevin Grumbach, Michael Drake, Karen Vranizan, Nicole Lurie, Dennis Keane, and Andrew B. Bindman. 1996. "The Role of Black and Hispanic Physicians in Providing Health Care for Underserved Populations." *New England Journal of Medicine* 334, no. 20: 1305–10.

Kosa, John, and Robert E. Coker. 1965. "The Female Physician in Public Health: Conflict and Reconciliation of the Professional and Sex Roles." *Sociology and Social Research* 49, no. 3: 294–305.

Kotelchuck, Ronda. 1994. "The New York City Health System: A Paradigm Under Siege." *Social Work in Ambulatory Care* 21, no. 1: 21–33.

Krause, Elliott A. 1971. *The Sociology of Occupations.* Boston: Little, Brown, and Company.

Kritzer, Herbert, and Carl N. Zimet. 1967. "A Retrospective View of Medical Specialty Choice." *Journal of Medical Education* 42 (January): 47–53.

Kusserow, R.P. 1992a. *Use of Emergency Rooms by Medicaid Recipients.* Washington, D.C.: Department of Health and Human Services, Office of the Inspector General.

————. 1992b. *Controlling Emergency Room Use: State Medicaid Reports.* Washington, D.C.: Department of Health and Human Services, Office of the Inspector General.

Langwell, Kathryn M. 1982. "Differences by Sex in Economic Returns Associated with Physician Specialization." *Journal of Health Politics, Policy and Law* 6, no. 4: 752–61.

Latour, Bruno, and Steve Woolgar. 1979. *Laboratory Life: The Social Construction of Scientific Facts.* Beverly Hills, CA: Sage.

Lenhart, Sharyn. 1993. "Gender Discrimination: A Health and Career Development Problem for Women Physicians." *Journal of the American Medical Association* 48, no.5: 155–59.

Levine, Donald N. 1977. "Simmel at a Distance: On the History and Systematics of the Sociology of the Stranger." *Sociological Focus* 10, no. 1: 15–29.

Lieberson, Stanley. 1958. "Ethnic Groups and the Practice of Medicine." *American Sociological Review* 23, no. 5: 542–49.

Lipson, Debra J. 1997. "Medicaid Managed Care and Community Providers: New Partnerships." *Health Affairs* 16 (July/August): 91–107.

Long, Stephen H., Russell F. Settle, and Bruce C. Stuart. 1986. "Reimbursement and Access to Physicians' Services Under Medicaid." *Journal of Health Economics* 5: 235–51.

Lorber, Judith. 1981. "The Limits of Sponsorship for Women Physicians." *Journal of the American Medical Association* 36, no.11: 329–38.

————. 1984. *Women Physicians Careers, Status, and Power.* New York: Tavistock Publications.

———. 1993. "Why Women Physicians Will Never Be True Equals in the American Medical Profession." Pp. 62–76 in *Gender, Work and Medicine*, ed. E. Riska, and K. Weger. London: Sage Publications.

Lorber, Judith, and Martha Ecker. 1983. "Career Development of Female and Male Physicians." *Journal of Medical Education* 58 (June): 447–56.

Lopate, Carol. 1968. *Women in Medicine*. Baltimore: Johns Hopkins Press.

Lyden, Fremont J., H. Jack Geiger, and Osler L. Peterson. 1968. *The Training of Good Physicians—Critical Factors in Career Choices*. Cambridge: Harvard University Press.

Madow, William G., Harold Nisselson, and Ingram Olkin., eds. 1983. *Incomplete Data in Sample Surveys, Volume 1: Report and Case Studies*. New York: Academic Press.

Managed Care Week. 1994. "Managed Medicaid Programs Serving 8 Million Recipients," 3 October.

Manheim, Larry M., Philip J. Held, and Judith Wooldrige. 1978. "Physician Acceptance of Medicaid Patients." *Staff Paper* SP–78B–02. Princeton: Mathmatica Policy Research.

Marshall, Robert J., John P. Fulton, and Albert F. Wessen. 1978. "Physician Career Outcomes and the Process of Medical Education." *Journal of Health and Social Behavior* 19: 124–38.

Martin, Patricia Yancey. 1982. "Fair Science: Test of Assertion? A Response to Cole's Women in Science." *Sociological Review* 30: 478–508.

Medicaid Access Study Group. 1994. "Access of Medicaid Recipients to Outpatient Care." *New England Journal of Medicine* 334, no. 20: 1426–30.

Merton, Robert K. 1957. *Social Theory and Social Structure*. New York: The Free Press.

———. 1968. "The Matthew Effect in Science." *Science* 159: 56–63.

———. 1973. *The Sociology of Science*. Chicago: University of Chicago Press.

Mick, Stephen S. 1987. "Sector Theory, Stratification, and Health Policy: Foreign and U.S. Medical Graduates in Medical Practice." *Journal of Health and Social Behavior* 28 (March): 74–88.

Mick, Stephen S., and Shoou–Yih Daniel Lee. 1997. "The Safety–Net Role of International Medical Graduates." *Health Affairs* 16 July/August): 141–50.

Miller, Alfred E. 1977. "The Changing Structure of the Medical Profession in Urban and Suburban Settings." *Social Science and Medicine* 11, no. 4: 233–43.

Miller, Stephen J. 1970. *Prescription for Leadership: Training for the Medical Elite*. Chicago: Aldine.

Mitchell, Janet B. 1983. "Medicaid Participation by Medical and Surgical Specialists." *Medical Care* 21, no. 9: 929–38.

———. 1991. "Physician Participation in Medicaid Revisited." *Medical Care* 29, no. 7: 645–53.

Mitchell, Janet B., and Jerry Cromwell. 1980. "Medicaid Mills: Fact or Fiction." *Health Care Financing Review* (summer): 37–49.

Mitchell, Janet B., and Rachel Schurman. 1984. "Access to Private Obstetrics/Gynecology Services Under Medicaid." *Medical Care* 22, no. 11: 1026–37.

Morantz–Sanchez, Regina M. 1985. *Sympathy and Science*. Oxford: Oxford University Press.

Mullan, Fitzhugh, Robert M. Politzer, and Howard Davis. 1995. "Medical Migration and the Physician Workforce." *Journal of the American Medical Association* 273, no. 19: 1521–27.

Mullan, Fitzhugh. 1996. "Powerful Hands: Making the Most of Graduate Medical Education." *Health Affairs* 15, no. 2: 250–53.

Mumford, Emily. 1970. *Interns: From Intern to Physician*. Cambridge, Mass.: Harvard University Press.

Myers, Cindi. 1995. "Different Paths, Same Goal— International Medical Graduates Struggle with Licensure Hurdles, Discrimination." *Texas Medicine* (February): 30–32.

Nadel, V. 1993. *Emergency Departments: Unevenly Affected by Growth and Change in Patient Use.* Washington, D.C.: General Accounting Office, Human Resources Division, (GAO/HRD publication no. 93–4).

Nadelson, Carol C. 1991. "Advancing Through the Medical Hierarchy." *Journal of the American Medical Association* 46, no. 3: 95–99.

Nager, Norma, and Frough Saadatmand. 1991. "The Status of Medical Education for Black Americans." *Journal of the National Medical Association* 83, no. 9: 787–92.

National Governors' Association. 1983. *A Catalogue of State Medicaid Program Changes.* Washington, D.C.: National Governors' Association.

Navarro, Vicente. 1995. "Why Congress Did Not Enact Health Care Reform." *Journal of Health Politics, Policy and Law* 20, no. 2: 455–62.

Nation's Health. 1995. "More Medicaid Patients in Managed Care Plans in 1994," January.

New York Times. 1993a. "Sensing a Loss of Control, More Doctors Call It Quits," 9 March, A1.

———. 1993b. "Clinton May Seek Lid on Doctor Fees and Liability Suits," 9 March, A1.

———. 1995. "G.O.P. Seeks Medicaid Overhaul, Giving Vast Authority to States," 1 April, 1.

———. 1995. "Young Doctors Find Specialist Jobs Hard to Get," 15 April, 1.

———. 1995. "Why Student Aid Matters," 6 June, A24.

Park, Robert E. 1928. "Human Migration and the Marginal Man." *American Journal of Sociology* 33, no. 6 (May): 881–93.

Pane, Gregg A., Michael C. Farner, and Kym A. Salness. 1991. "Health Care Access Problems of Medically Indigent Emergency Department Walk-in Patients." *Annals of Emergency Medicine* 20, no. 7: 730–33.

Perloff, Janet D. 1996. "Medicaid Managed Care and Urban Poor People: Implications for Social Work." *Health and Social Work* 20: 181–95.

Perloff, Janet D., Phillip R. Kletke, and Kathryn M. Neckerman. 1986. "Recent Trends in Pediatrician Participation in Medicaid." *Medical Care* 24, no. 8: 749–60.

———. 1987a. *Medicaid and Pediatric Primary Care.* Baltimore: Johns Hopkins University Press.

———. 1987b. "Physicians' Decision to Limit Medicaid Participation: Determinants and Policy Implications." *Journal of Health Politics, Policy and Law* 12, no. 2: 221–35.

Petersdorf, Robert G. 1990. "From the President." *Academic Medicine* 65: 29.

———. 1992. "Not a Choice, an Obligation." *Academic Medicine* 67, no. 2: 73–79.

Petersdorf, Robert G., Kathleen S. Turner, Herbert W. Nickens, and Timothy Ready. 1990. "Minorities in Medicine: Present and Future." *Academic Medicine* November 65, no. 11: 663–70.

Peterson, Stephen E., and Carlson, Paul. 1992. "Mentorship Program for Minority Students." *Academic Medicine* 67, no. 8: 521.

Pew Health Professions Commission. 1995. *Critical Challenges: Revitalizing the Health Professions for the Twenty–first Century: Third Report of the Pew Health Professions Commission* San Francisco: University of California at San Francisco Center for the Health Professions.

Physician Payment Review Commission (PPRC). 1990. *Annual Report to Congress.* Washington, D.C.

———. 1991. *Annual Report to Congress.* Washington, D.C.

Pinn–Wiggins,Vivian W. 1985. "An Affirmation of Minorities in Medicine." *New England Journal of Medicine* 313, no. 24: 1540–41.

Reskin, Barbara F. 1978. "Sex Differentiation and the Social Organization of Science." *Sociological Inquiry* 48, no. 3: 3–37.

———. 1988. "Bringing the Men Back In: Sex Differentiation and the Devaluation of Women's Work." *Gender and Society* 2: 58–81.

Richard, Michel Paul. 1969. "The Negro Physician: Babbitt or Revolutionary?" *Journal of Health and Social Behavior* 10 (December): 265–74.

Riley, Trish. 1995. "Medicaid: The Role of the States." *Journal of the American Medical Association* 274, no. 3: 267–70.

Rinke, Carlotta M. 1981a. "The Economic and Academic Status of Women Physicians." *Journal of the American Medical Association* 245, no. 22: 2305–6.

Rinke, Carlotta M. 1981b. "The Professional Identities of Women Physicians." *Journal of the American Medical Association* 245, no. 23: 2419–21.

Rivo, Marc L., and David Satcher. 1993. "Improving Access to Health Care Through Physician Workforce Reform." *Journal of the American Medical Association* 270, no. 9: 1074–78.

Rosenbaum, Sara. 1997. "A Look Inside Medicaid Managed Care." *Health Affairs* 16 (July/August): 266–71.

Rowland, Diana. 1993. "Health Care of the Poor: The Contribution of Social Insurance." Pp. 107–24 in *Medical Care and the Health of the Poor,* ed. D.E.Rogers, and E. Ginzberg. Boulder, CO: Westview Press.

———. 1994. "Lessons from the Medicaid Experience." Pp. 190–207 in *Critical Issues in U.S. Health Reform,* ed. E. Ginzberg. Boulder, Colo.: Westview Press.

———. 1995. "Medicaid at 30." *Journal of the American Medical Association* 274, no. 3: 271–73.

Rowland, Diana, Barbara Lyons, and Jennifer Edwards. 1988. "Medicaid: Health Care for the Poor in the Reagan Era." *Annual Review of Public Health* 9: 427–50.

Rowland, Diana, and K. Hanson. 1996. "Medicaid: Moving to Managed Care." *Health Affairs* (fall): 150–52.

Schauffler, Helen Halpin, and Jessica Wolin. 1996. "Community Health Clinics under Managed Competition: Navigating Uncharted Waters." *Journal of Health Politics, Policy and Law* 21, no. 3: 461–88.

Schermerhorn, Gerry R., Jerry A. Colliver, Steven J. Verhulst, and Ellen L. Schmidt. 1986. "Factors that Influence Career Patterns of Women Physicians." *Journal of the American Medical Women's Association* 41, no. 3: 74–78.

Schwartz, Anne, David C. Colby, and Anne Lenhard Reisinger. 1991. "Variation in Medicaid Physician Fees." *Health Affairs* (spring): 131–39.

Schwartzbaum, Allan M., John H. McGrath, and Robert A. Rothman. 1973. "The Perception of Prestige Differences among Medical Subspecialties." *Social Science and Medicine* 7, no. 5: 365–71.

Shea, Steven, and Mindy Thompson Fullilove. 1985. "Entry of Black and Other Minority Students into U.S. Medical Schools." *New England Journal of Medicine* 313, no. 15: 933–40.

Shesser, Robert , Thomas Kirsch, Jeff Smith, and Robert Hirsch. 1991. "An Analysis of Emergency Department Use by Patients with Minor Illness." *Annals of Emergency Medicine* 20, no. 7: 743–48.

Shortell, Stephen M. 1974. "Occupational Prestige Differences Within the Medical and Allied Health Professions." *Social Science and Medicine* 8, no. 1: 1–9.

Shuval, Judith T. 1985. "Social Functions of Medical Licensing: A Case Study of Soviet Immigrant Physicians in Israel." *Social Science and Medicine* 20, no. 9: 901–9.

Silverstein, Gail. 1997. "Physicians' Perceptions of Commercial and Medicaid Managed Care Plans: A Comparison." *Journal of Health Politics, Policy and Law* 22, no. 1: 5–21.

Sirridge, Marjorie S. 1985. "The Mentor System in Medicine—How It Works for Women." *Journal of the American Medical Women's Association* 40, no. 2: 51–53.

Sloan, Frank, Jerry Cromwell, and Janet Mitchell. 1978. *Private Physicians and Public Programs.* Lexington, Mass: D.C. Heath and Company.

Slotkin, J.S. 1943. "The Status of the Marginal Man." *Sociology and Social Research* 28, no. 1: 47–54.

Solomon, David N. 1961. "Ethnic and Class Differences Among Hospitals as Contingencies in Medical Careers." *American Journal of Sociology* 66, no. 5: 463–71.

Sparer, Michael. 1996. "Medicaid Managed Care and the Health Reform Debate: Lessons from New York and California." *Journal of Health Politics, Policy and Law* 21, no. 3: 433–60.

Sparer, Michael. 1997. "Laboratories and the Health Care Marketplace: The Limits of State Workforce Policy." *Journal of Health Politics, Policy and Law* 22, no. 3: 789–814.

Starr, Paul. 1982. *The Social Transformation of American Medicine.* New York: Basic Books.

———. 1986. "Health Care for the Poor: the Past Twenty Years." Pp. 106–32 in *Fighting Poverty: What Works and What Doesn't,* ed. S.H. Danziger, and D.H. Weinberg. Cambridge, Mass: Harvard University Press.

Steinbrook, Robert. 1996. "Diversity in Medicine." *New England Journal of Medicine* 334, no. 20: 1327–28.

Stern, Bernhard J. 1958. "The Specialist and the General Practitioner." Pp. 352–60 in *Patients, Physicians and Illness: Source Book in Behavioral Science and Medicine,* ed. E.C. Jaco. Glencoe: The Free Press.

Stevens, Robert, and Rosemary Stevens. 1974. *Welfare Medicine in America: A Case Study of Medicaid.* New York: Free Press.

Stevens, Rosemary, Louis Wolf Goodman, and Stephen S. Mick. 1978. *The Alien Doctors.* New York: John Wiley & Sons.

Stimmel, Barry D. 1996. "Congress and the International Medical Graduate." *Mount Sinai Journal of Medicine* 63, nos. 5 and 6: 359–63.

Stonequist, Everett V. 1935. "The Problem of the Marginal Man." *American Journal of Sociology* 61, no. 1: 1–12.

———. 1961. *The Marginal Man* New York: Russell & Russell.

Sudit, Myriam. 1987. *Ideology or Self-Interest? Medical Students' Attitudes Toward National Health Insurance.* Ph.D. diss., Columbia University.

Tan, Kong Meng. 1977. "Foreign Medical Graduate Performance–A Review." *Medical Care* 15, no. 10: 822–29.

Taylor, Robert E., James C. Hunt, and Patra B. Temple. 1990. "Recruiting Black Medical Students: A Decade of Effort." *Academic Medicine* 65, no. 5: 279–88.

Tesch, Bonnie J., Helen M. Wood, Amy L. Helwig, and Ann Butler Nattinger. 1995. "Promotion of Women Physicians in Academic Medicine: Glass Ceiling or Sticky Floor?" *Journal of the American Medical Association* 273, no. 13: 1022–25.

Thurmond, Vera B., and Antonio Mott. 1990. "Minority Students' Career Choices and Education Five Years After They Completed a Summer Enrichment Program." *Academic Medicine* 65, no. 7: 478–79.

Torrey, E. Fuller and Robert L. Taylor. 1973. "Cheap Labor From Poor Nations." *American Journal of Psychiatry* 130, no. 4: 428–34.

Tuchman, Gaye. 1980. "Discriminating Science." *Social Policy* 11 (May–June): 59–64.

U.S. Bureau of the Census. 1991. *Poverty in the United States: 1990.* Current Population Reports, Series P–60, No. 175.

U.S. Department of Commerce, Economics and Statistics Administration, Bureau of the Census. 1994. *1990 Decennial Census of Population and Housing* on CD–ROM, Washington, D.C.

U.S. Department of Health, Education and Welfare (USDHEW). 1975. "History and Evolution of Medicaid." Pp. 5–10 in *Medicaid: Lessons for National Health Insurance,* ed. A. D. Spiegel, and S. Podair. Rockville, Md.: Aspen Systems Corporation.

U. S. Department of Health and Human Services (USDHHS). 1983. *Non–Urgent Use of Hospital Emergency Departments by Medicaid and Medicare Beneficiaries.* Office of the Inspector General, Washington, D.C.: U.S. Government Printing Office.

———. 1985. *Report of the Secretary's Task Force on Black and Minority Health.* Washington, D.C.: U.S. Government Printing Office.

———. 1990a. *Minorities & Women in the Health Fields.* Washington, D.C.: U.S. Government Printing Office.

———. 1990b. *Education of Physicians to Improve Access to Care for the Underserved: Proceedings from the Second HRSA Primary Care Conference.* (21–23 March).

———. Health Care Financing Administration. 1992. *Medicaid Statistics: Program and Financial Statistics Fiscal Year 1990.* Washington, D.C.: U.S. Government Printing Office.

———. 1993. *Minority Physicians: A Profile.* Washington, D.C.: U.S. Government Printing Office.

Walsh, Mary Roth. 1977. *Doctors Wanted: No Women Need Apply Sexual Barriers in the Medical Profession, 1835–1975.* New Haven: Yale University.

Watts, Velma Gibson, Catherine T. Harris, and Willie Pearson. 1989. "Course Selections and Career Plans of Black Participants in a Summer Intervention Program for Minority Students." *Academic Medicine* 64, no. 3: 166–67.

Weisman, Carol S., David M. Levine, Donald M. Steinwachs, and Gary A. Chase. 1980. "Male and Female Physician Career Patterns: Specialty Choices and Graduate Training." *Journal of Medical Education* 55 (October): 813–25.

Westling–Wikstrand, Helena, Mary A. Monk, and Caroline Bedell–Thomas. 1970. "Some Characteristics Related to the Career Status of Women Physicians." *Hopkins Medical Journal* 127 (November): 273–86.

Willie, Charles Vert. 1975. *Oreo: On Race and Marginal Men and Women.* Wakefield, Mass.: Parameter Press.

Wilson, Donald E., and Jeanette M. Kaczmarek. 1993. "The History of African–American Physicians and Medicine in the United States." *Journal of the Association for Academic Minority Phyicians* (4 July) no. 3: 93–98.

Xu, Gang, Susan L. Rattner, J. Jon Veloski, Mohammadreza Hojat, Sylvia K. Fields, and Barbara Barzansky. 1995. "A National Study of the Factors Influencing Men and Women Physicians' Choices of Primary Care Specialties." *Academic Medicine* 70, no. 5: 398–404.

Yudkowsky, Beth K., Jenifer D.C. Cartland, and Samuel S. Flint. 1990. "Pediatrician Participation in Medicaid: 1978 to 1989." *Pediatrics* 85, no. 4: 567–77.

Zuckerman, Harriet. 1977. *Scientific Elite: Nobel Laureates in theUnited States.* New York: Free Press.

Index